MW01036912

# BEAUTIFUL
# UNIQUE
# FACES

## ANITA EAST

**Copyright © Anita East**
First published in Australia in 2020
by Karen McDermott
Waikiki, WA 6169

All rights reserved. No part of this book may be used or reproduced by any means, graphic, electronic, or mechanical, including photocopying, recording, taping or by any information storage retrieval system without the written permission of the copyright owner except in the case of brief quotations embodied in critical articles and reviews. Although the author and publisher have made every effort to ensure that the information in this book was correct at press time, the author and publisher do not assume and hereby disclaim any liability to any party for any loss, damage, or disruption caused by errors or omissions, whether such errors or omissions result from negligence, accident, or any other cause. This book is not intended as a substitute for the medical advice of physicians. The reader should regularly consult a physician in matters relating to his/her health and particularly with respect to any symptoms that may require diagnosis or medical attention.

Cover Design: Nada Backovic
Interior design: Ida Jansson
Editor: Louisa Deasey
Editor: Anjanette Fennell
Editor: Dannielle Line
Proofread: Carolyn De Ridder

National Library of Australia Catalogue-in-Publication data:
Beautiful Unique Faces/Anita East
Success/Self-help

ISBN: 978-0-6489123-0-9 (sc)
ISBN: 978-0-6489123-1-6 (e)

*This book is dedicated to Agatha and Daisy.*
*May you always know how Beautiful and Unique your Faces are.*

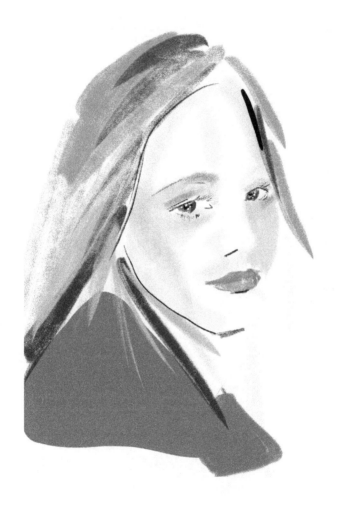

My daughter Agatha.

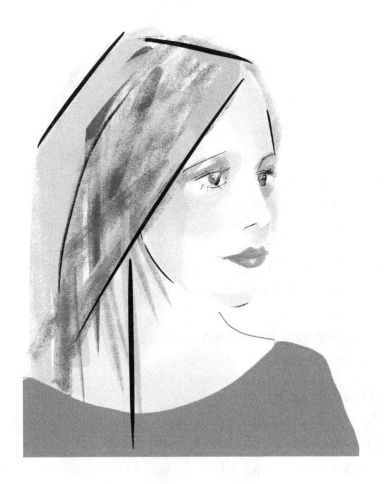

**My daughter Daisy.**

# Contents

# Introduction

# WHY I NEEDED TO WRITE THIS BOOK.

As a leading cosmetic injectable and aesthetic medicine specialist with a busy private clinic in Brisbane, I've treated over 18,000 clients. The first nurse practitioner in Brisbane to specialise in cosmetic medicine and skin, I have a background that combines international stage and screen performing with cosmetic medicine. This gives me a unique, empathetic perspective to women wishing to enhance their facial features.

After foundational studies in cardiac and skin medicine, I moved to the United Kingdom, where I studied opera and acting at the prestigious English National Opera and the Royal Central School of Speech and Drama. I worked as a TV Presenter for Sky Sports, the BBC and UK breakfast television. I was a successful stage and screen actress in the UK and Australia with stints on *The Bill, Neighbours, Offspring, Rush*, and various TV commercials, West End Theatre productions, and feature films.

On one of these films, my purpose crystallised. On a film set in London sixteen years ago in the hair and makeup department,

I overheard a tense conversation between the director and the makeup artist. The lead actress turned up on the first day of the film shoot with grossly overfilled lips and a frozen, expressionless face. She was known for her stunning eyes, but now that her lips were so oddly shaped and large, her eyes were no longer as pretty as they'd once been.

The lead actress, the director, and the whole cast and crew, including myself, were heartbroken. The lead actress probably ruined the best chance she had of launching her acting career. And the film would likely be a flop given her inability to portray the story and show a true connection. But she'd done it because she believed she would look better if her lines were erased and her lips plumped. I vowed on that day to make it better. To somehow make cosmetic injectables look natural rather than scary and overdone, which thanks to reality TV was becoming all the rage. I set out on my mission as soon as the film shoot wrapped six weeks later. I'm a perfectionist and a people-pleaser by nature.

When I saw the pain that an actress's frozen, plumped up face caused, it's not surprising I felt compelled to research the perfect Botox treatment and make everything better. I was born into the role. What I didn't expect to find during this journey over the next sixteen years, was the secret to our beauty is right in front of our faces. And it has nothing to do with having something injected into or done to ourselves.

## The dangerous trend needs to stop now!

In writing this book, I'm speaking out against this common and hugely worrying trend. I'm putting myself at risk of being bullied, ostracised, hated, abused and shamed. Not only am I putting my family at risk of financial ruin because my business could be impacted, but I'm at risk of damaging myself. However, the call to head the change, start the movement and lead the way comes not just from my experiences but from hearing yours. The eighty patients I see every week, the women and men I speak to in passing and the conversations with my six teenage nieces all have something in common. They all tell me about the pressure they feel to look a certain way. And the women on my TV and social media pages are crying for help. I can't sleep at night, knowing the stuff I know and not doing my very best to make the world a safer and more accepting place for my two darling daughters. I'll continue to fight the good fight to ensure that they don't succumb to the social epidemic to become Pretty Ugly Faces.

## A word on Pretty Ugly Faces.

Pretty Ugly Face or PUF is a term coined by a patient of mine during a passionate discussion of why women were overtreating their faces with Botox and dermal fillers. It refers to the puffy, expressionless and unmoving face of someone who has had too much 'work' done or the wrong kind. Almost plastic in appearance, it results from striving for a perfected computer-generated shape, of filters and Facetune, of cartoon proportions and a wax-like look that is distinctly unnatural.

Pretty Ugly Faces refers to faces that have become almost too pretty, so that now they look ugly. Often the PUFs we see on our social media feed aren't even real. However, thanks to their celebrity following and the perfect features shown in these photos, women and men are fooled into thinking, to be happy, they too need to aspire to this impossible and non-human ideal.

## Call out the fraud.

Thankfully, social media accounts now exist with the sole purpose of exposing the media outlets and celebrities who fraudulently distort real images into heavily filtered ones. By showing their audience what the celebrity looks like in real life, side by side with their heavily filtered image, there is hope we can remove some pressure women or men feel to look like dolls.

## All women are beautiful.

I love all women. I've never met a woman who wasn't breathtakingly beautiful in her unique way. Sadly though, and in my experience, most women don't know what their unique beauty is. They've become so stuck in finding their beauty through the expectations of those around them, through what media and society set as the current beauty 'standard', they're at risk of losing their beauty forever.

## Why do we do it to ourselves?

The importance of your Unique Facial Feature will become more evident with every woman's story you read in my book; however, let me introduce you to its significance.

The overdone faces you know, see on TV, social media, and in the press...think hard about them. Would you describe them as beautiful? Can you describe something beautiful and unique about them? It's hard, isn't it? That's because when we become 'over-treated' (by that I mean overfilled and over-frozen) we lose our intrinsic beauty. I've had thousands of patients ask me why women do it to themselves. They seek answers from me. It's hard to explain why they do it, but I'm surrounded by it, and it's as simple as; they don't know what their Unique Facial Feature is, so they don't realise what makes them beautiful. If we don't know that we look good in green and everyone is wearing red, we will wear red, too. We don't know what we don't know. We take guidance from those we think are in the know—mainstream media, social media, friends, family. And we're always looking outside of ourselves for the answers we so cleverly have inside of us.

## Be the best *you* can be. Live *your* best life.

Sadly, women who are over-treated never believe they look good. Although they can look in the mirror and say;

*"Yes, my eyelashes are the best they can be." "My eyes are the best they can be." "My nose is the best it can be." "My lips are the best they can be." "My cheeks, the best they can be." "My jaw angle, yes, it's the best it can be." "My chin is the best it can be." "My frown, forehead, crow's feet are the best they can be." "My hair, my breasts, my body, my clothes, my accessories are all the best they can be." "I'm winning at life."*

Seldom do they feel satisfied and so the cycle of continually believing something is wrong with their face continues. They see another set of lips or another jawline they want, so they have more and more done until they're unrecognisable.

The illusion of perfection are the standards set out by celebrities and influencers. If every single feature on your face is the most 'perfect' it can be, your perfected face no longer stands out for any reason other than looking 'weird.'

You'll read in Chapter One **how over-treated faces fade into insignificance and can even appear unattractive.**

A flower that has the following is almost comical rather than real: Giant, brightly coloured petals, an extravagant stamen with elaborate projections, a wondrous stem with giant brilliant too-green leaves and an incredible scent that knocks you over when you come close. More suited to a child's drawing or piece of abstract artwork, can it indeed be taken seriously? The over-treated face is similar. Almost doll-like, over-treated faces look odd and not human. They're almost machine-like and it's hard to make a connection.

## Do the next right thing.

Over the last few years, my moral code has been at odds with my sense of responsibility for contributing to a society in crisis which continually seeks perfect facial features. I took my role as a protector of my patients extremely seriously. As a clinician and contributor to this epidemic, I felt it was my responsibility to ensure they didn't get sucked into the rabbit hole of over-treated faces too.

In August 2019, I nearly died from a fatal asthma attack. I'd become incredibly unwell, but was so determined not to let my patients down that I didn't rest or slow down in the leading months. Adamant I could do it all, I tried to please my patients, whose demands were growing exponentially. But I was losing the battle of keeping their expectations realistic when the world of filtered social media was telling them to be happy, they *needed* to have the lips, cheeks, jaw, chin, and frozen face. When they didn't become more joyful as social media promised, I felt responsible.

Even while I was losing consciousness during my asthma attack, I was only thinking about the patients booked in to see me that day and how I couldn't possibly let them down by dying. I should've been thinking about my husband and my daughters, but no, I was thinking about how, if I died, I'd let my patients down. How insane is that? I put them and the pursuit of perfection above my own life.

While working on my second draft of this book, I started talking with a bestselling author who helped me workshop the book's premise.

I told her I was writing a non-fiction book about my profession: cosmetic medicine, in particular the rise of Botox and dermal fillers. Her first response was to say she wasn't my ideal reader, but she'd help me as much as she could, given her limited experience or interest in cosmetic enhancements. By the end of our session, she'd shifted entirely. She said she'd been wrong, that she was my ideal reader. Although Botox and dermal fillers may not be something she'd ever imagined having, she said she was a woman first, so of course she wanted to know the secret to looking beautiful. Now that I'd revealed to her the secret of being her most beautiful, she felt like all the pieces fell into place of the mystery to her personal beauty. Suddenly, it all made sense. She anticipated the day this book would hit the shelves saying, "Anita, the world needs your book."

## Is this book for you?

I have a mix of women who come into my practice and I expect, I will have the same mix of women reading this book. Those who worry if they have a treatment, they will look overdone and 'frozen' like the women they see on their TV and social media pages. And those who worry I'll tell them there is nothing I can do for them and they're beyond saving. Those whose faces are already over-frozen and overfilled but still want more injected. And, finally, those who have been educated about their beautiful, unique facial feature and have the balance right. A bit like when Goldilocks found baby bear's porridge.

## It can be *'just right.'*

I want you to feel like Goldilocks with her perfect porridge when you've finished this book. You'll know exactly what you should and shouldn't be highlighting on your face, how to know when enough is enough, and how to 'support' the major players in your beautiful, unique face. Because that's what you have: a beautiful and unique face.

Get ready to meet some of the amazing women I've met in my life. Their stories have taught me the secrets of discovering breathtaking beauty and happiness. Some of their stories are heartbreaking and they don't end well. Others are empowering and are the Unique Facial Features version of fairy tales. All will teach you valuable lessons and, like all good fables, how to avoid evil (keep yourself safe) through tales of woe, as well as how to empower yourself to look, feel and be your absolute best.

Each of the women you meet in Beautiful Unique Faces have been given a fictional name. Their stories are comprised of many of the women I have met throughout my career. No case study will be recognisable as relating to one woman. Each case study tells the story of all women.

I've written this book for all the women in the world who've ever felt unhappy with their appearance. You're not alone. My book will teach you how to love your face (or fall in love with it once more). I've also written this book for all of us in the service industry, whose hope is to make women feel good about themselves. You're not alone, either. If you hope to make women feel better about themselves, this book is also for you.

This book will empower you on how to uncover what is most beautiful about you. This book is for all women. This book is for you.

Together we are stronger.
Together we can make a difference to all the
girls and women we know and love.
Together we can feel safe leaning into
vulnerability and leaning away from perfection.

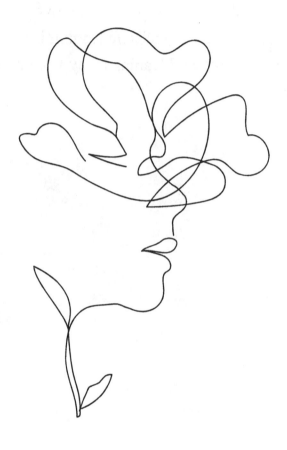

# Chapter One

## Part One

## WHY DO OUR FACIAL FEATURES MATTER SO MUCH?

When we remove all facial movement, we remove the ability to show vulnerability, and vulnerability is what nurtures connection in human relationships. When we remove all facial movement, it creates a significant impact on our life and our relationships.

CASE STUDY: JUSTINE

### "I want all my facial movements gone."

Justine was a patient at the practice I was working at during the start of my career. Although I have treated thousands of women since Justine, I think about her often. I wonder if there was more I could've done to help her. No, that's not correct, I know there was more I could've done to help her. Justine is a lesson to us all.

*"I want all my facial movements gone. I don't want my husband or children knowing how I'm feeling."*

*Justine had a 'hard' look to her face, and I was confused and put off by her steely reserve. I was a novice injector. I thought Justine was joking when she said she wanted all of her facial movements gone.*

*I joined in on her joke and laughed, but was met with stony silence. Justine was serious. She made me nervous. I excused myself and sought advice from my boss, who confirmed that Justine always took more than the maximum dose. It was usual for her to want to be completely expressionless.*

*I treated Justine with the doses she'd received throughout the three years previously. Twelve weeks later, Justine returned for her next treatment, with the same request: "I want all my facial movements gone. I don't want my husband or children knowing how I'm feeling," and, again, I treated her with the same doses. It was the last time I managed Justine as I moved to another of the Doctor's clinics. This time I asked Justine why she needed to hide her feelings.*

*"I do this to protect my children. So, they can't see how unhappy I am."*

From a large family, Justine married her high school sweetheart young and started a family early. Her husband, a loving and attentive father to their three children, adored Justine.

After the birth of her first child, Justine suffered from post-natal depression. Rather than seeking help, which in the early 2000s wasn't as accepted as today, she decided to have another child to see if her depression 'would go away.' But it didn't. It became worse with each pregnancy and birth.

Her husband, the new young CEO of a successful company,

was excelling in his career. He relied on the image of his perfect family unit to seal lucrative deals with other businessmen who held high family values.

*"It's a complicated system, but it works. There is no room for me to be ill."*

Justine understood her responsibility and, rather than seeking treatment for her mental health which she suspected she might need, she elected instead to hide her emotions, hoping to squash down her pain. She found that by removing her ability to look sad, angry, distraught, or depressed, she wore a proverbial mask that hid how she was truly feeling. Justine and her practitioners, including myself, didn't consider the negative impact that frozen facial features and an inability to show her true feelings would have on her relationship with her husband, her children and, ultimately, herself.

*"Our first argument about it was on the way home from a dinner with an important client and his wife. My husband said I was cold, and that I hadn't tried hard enough to be friends with the man's wife. But that night I was trying especially hard to be happy and attentive."*

It made no sense to Justine. Convinced that her depression was seeping through her frozen face, rather than seeking professional psychological help, she increased the quantity of her treatments.

## It's all about connection.

When we approach someone, regardless of whether we know them, we look at their face to check it's safe to approach. Our face is how people know our mood and our feelings. It's the quickest way to identify a potential 'threat' from another human being.

When someone first looks at you, they aren't looking at your hair, figure or clothes to establish if you're safe to approach. They're looking at your face. You could dress in gorgeous clothing, but if you have a big frown plastered across your face, people will think twice about approaching you. Similarly, if you have a big smile on your face and your smile is a warm and genuine smile, people will assume you're safe to approach.

An emotionless face, devoid of both negative and positive emotion characteristics, is hard to warm to. People will tread cautiously with someone they can't read and assume now isn't a good time to approach them.

Let me break it down for you. Humans seek approval and love from others. We do this by connecting with others. We need to connect with other people, so we feel like we belong. Only when we feel like we belong, can we truly feel safe and calm.

Babies connect in the only way they're able, through physical touch. If babies aren't touched, they can't feel safe, and they can't feel loved. And as horrible as this is to write, babies can stop growing due to a lack of physical touch, and if this continues, they can die.

We literally thrive on connection. Do you know the people with whom you instantly connect? As soon as you think about them and see them, you feel loved and accepted. We need to be accepted. It's what enables us to grow and flourish.

---

Vulnerability = Connection = Safety = Love

---

## Facial expression allows us to connect.

When we interact with others, we show a range of emotions that help the other person to interpret and respond to us accordingly.

If we're telling the other person a sad story, yet we're showing no signs of the sadness we feel, it's confusing for our audience. They are not sure if we're as sad, angry or desperate as we say we are because we're not showing the emotion that reflects what we're feeling. This disconnect leads to a lack of trust.

Equally, if someone is saying they're upset about their pet who is unwell, but doesn't show it, we think the story isn't true or that what the person says is contrary to what they feel.

Think about the actress who turned up on day one of the film shoot and couldn't show the emotional range necessary of her character's harrowing story—the loss of a child. The film's audience needed to see the pain she was suffering to enable their connection to her, to her story and, ultimately, to the film. But with frozen facial expressions, it was impossible.

The actor who doesn't seem genuine in their portrayal of a character's emotion can be written off as a 'bad actor.' We can switch off – it's not personal. Yet the person with too much Botox in their face who can't portray their feelings genuinely, is deemed untrustworthy. This is what I want to stop in our society. And this book teaches us how.

## Storytelling connects us.

We love to be moved. Other people's stories move us and, equally, our stories move other people. We need to empathise with those around us to create connection with them. If we're the person seeking connection, but can't express our feelings through our facial expressions because they're frozen, we come away feeling misunderstood. It makes us feel disconnected and alone.

So, what happens when we completely erase the lines in our face that tell our story or allow us to show our story?

At rest (and by this, I mean when we're merely being and not portraying any emotion at all) it can make us look cold and aloof. Think of the reality TV stars who say one thing yet show another (or nothing at all). The only way we can know how they're feeling is through the words they're saying rather than what their face is showing.

Frozen facial expressions make it impossible for us to connect with others. People will perceive us as inauthentic. If we can't be read, others feel safer keeping us at arm's length.

When we're moving and animating, telling our story and interacting with others, if our facial features represent what we're saying, they can't help but connect.


## JUSTINE CONTINUED.

Justine thought her marriage was showing signs of strain. She and her husband weren't communicating well anymore and, as a result, she was feeling isolated and even more unhappy.

Over the next twelve months, Justine had increasingly extensive treatments on her face. After every treatment, she felt really good.

*"It was almost like I feel like I've had an injection of happy juice or something. I just feel happy for the first few days. It's so lovely. It's addictive," Justine said.*

*She continued, "I'd examine each feature on my face to see what looked imperfect. Then at my appointment I'd tell the injector what I wanted to be done."*

By isolating each feature of her face, Justine could keep track of what she felt she needed 'fixed'. It gave her a sense of control she was missing in other areas of her life.

Justine had her lips plumped, her cheeks filled, her chin filled, and her jaw sharpened. She had her frown and forehead lines erased, and her crow's feet all but removed.

Justine's unique facial feature were her unusual looking, wide-set, hazel-coloured eyes. With each treatment she had, though, her eyes lost focus, and her lips, jaw, or cheeks took centre stage.

Justine told me that, during this period, her relationship with her children and husband became very strained. Her husband even told her he didn't know who she was anymore. He accused her of not caring about them and yelled, "You don't even look like you, I mean who the hell are you anyway?"

Justine felt she was growing more distant from them, and regardless of how she tried to show them how much she loved and cared for them, they didn't believe her.

Her husband moved out, and their children split their time between her and her husband. It was devastating to both Justine and her husband. They'd always valued their marriage and the stability of their family for their children.

Over the next twelve months, as the full force of their marriage separation took hold, Justine reduced the frequency and quantity of her treatments.

I caught up with Justine at this time, two years after I'd last treated her. I almost didn't recognise her. She looked vulnerable, and I know this sounds strange, but she looked real. In complete contrast to how I felt when I first met Justine, my heart immediately warmed to her.

Justine was seeing a psychologist for her post-natal depression, and she and her husband were having counselling to heal their marriage. They were communicating better than they'd done for a long time.

*"I think it's going to be ok," she told me.*

*She smiled and, in that instant, her unusual eyes crinkled up softly, and she looked genuinely hopeful and happy.*

We decided on a subtle treatment, half the doses she'd been having in the years before. We established a plan to make her beautiful, unique eyes the lead actor of her face and only treat the parts of her face that allowed her eyes to express their warmth and vulnerability fully.

Vulnerability nurtures joy, growth, and love, and Justine had lacked this in her life for quite some time.

## We're most beautiful when we're most human.

Sadly, this case study has an unhappy ending, which I won't share. The message I want Justine's story to teach you, dear reader, is that you are most beautiful when you are most human. We can't use Botox or dermal fillers (just as we can't use alcohol, drugs, food, or exercise) to treat a heart and mind that needs healing. Yes, we can use Botox or dermal fillers as a healthy accompaniment to our life - to improve how we feel about ourselves and the way we look. Yet give it any more responsibility than that and you're headed for a terrible shock, like dear Justine.

CASE STUDY: STELLA

## "I felt like it not only changed my smile, but I couldn't smile at all."

Stella came to me as a last resort. Not entirely new to treatments, she'd had Botox injected into her crow's feet once before.

Stella had been at a dinner party the month before, when as it often does, the topic of Botox came up. One guest helpfully suggested Stella needed to have some treatment. "You have wrinkles around your eyes, you can get rid of those with Botox," the guest pointed out.

Stella felt the last time she'd had Botox, it changed her smile.

*"I didn't like the way it made me look. I'm worried about having it done again. I felt like it not only changed my smile, but I couldn't smile at all," she told me.*

Stella had lovely eyes at rest, yes, but when she smiled is when they truly lit up. When she smiled, her whole face looked radiant. You wanted Stella to be your friend, and you wanted to spend as much time as you could with her, especially when she smiled. You know the kind of eyes I mean. Think George Clooney, Ryan Gosling. Their eyes are warm and inviting. Often when someone with eyes like Stella's smiles at you, you can't help but smile back.

*"It's weird, I had my crow's feet treated originally because the wrinkles were getting me down, but after I'd done it, I just felt sad," Stella said.*

Stella found that the treatment had the opposite effect to what she'd hoped she would experience. Her husband and others continually asked her if she was all right. Of course, the real reason they were asking was because Stella wasn't smiling anymore. And her eyes lost their sparkle.

## Behaviour breeds behaviour.

I'll say it a lot throughout the following chapters: behaviour breeds behaviour. If we look like there's something wrong with us and someone is treating us like something's wrong, almost by magic, we *feel* like something is wrong.

I hear it from my patients all the time. It's often the instigating reason they're sitting in my clinic. They've had a conversation that goes something like this:

> *"You look tired, are you ok?"*
> *"Really? I'm not tired, I'm sleeping well at the moment."*
> *"Ok, but you look tired. Is anything on your mind?"*
> *"No, I'm good."*
> *"Ok, I believe you."*

Now they have serious doubts whether they're ok. The way they're looking doesn't align with what they're feeling or what they're saying.

Think about how easily we misinterpret written text. Imagine how easily our face can be misread... especially if we're not showing the emotion that supports the words that we're saying.

Stella had this same experience from having the wrong treatment done. Her husband, who knew she'd had Botox in her crow's feet, didn't suspect the treatment was responsible for her feeling low. He was convinced there was something wrong with her and was worried he'd upset her. Soon Stella felt sad all the time and that perhaps there was something wrong with her.

A hairdresser, Stella, even had clients ask her if she was ok. Stella knew something was wrong then, but she still couldn't put her finger on it. She felt down and even saw her GP, who did blood tests which confirmed she was fit, well, and healthy.

## Facial Emotion Muscles - FEMs

As we've now learned from Justine and Stella, it's common to be misinterpreted when our facial emotion muscles or FEMs are frozen. In an ideal world, we'd soften the lines with Botox, rather than completely eradicate them.

The facial lines that depict negative emotions are our frown lines (which depict anger), our forehead lines (which depict worry), and our mouth frown (which depicts sadness). It's not wrong to portray these emotions. Contrary to popular belief, it's these emotions that allow us to connect with others.

The concern is when the wrinkles caused by these negative emotions remain etched into the skin and become static lines, meaning the negative-looking wrinkles are on our faces all the time. The same stands for hollows beneath the eyes called tear troughs and volume loss in our face, which leads to the jowls and a sunken and sorry look on our face. So, we may in fact be feeling happy but look cranky, sad or even scared.

Behaviour breeds behaviour. If we're perceived as being cranky, sad or scared, others will mirror the same behaviour back. Yet if we have frozen and distorted FEMs from too much Botox or dermal fillers and look distant and cold, we will be met with the same back. The more frozen our FEMs, the more likely that we're heading down the PUF rabbit hole.

## Over-frozen and overfilled isn't beautiful.

This sounds frightening, but the more frozen and distorted our FEMs, the higher the chance we'll experience greater isolation and relationship breakdowns. All from an inability to fully connect with others and, therefore, ourselves.

I've seen the impact it has when treatments are poorly performed. It can destroy relationships. Society has got it wrong. Over-frozen and overfilled isn't beautiful. As a clinician, I agree, it's a delicate balance to get 100% right. But it's worth understanding completely and being brave enough to be comfortable with your natural expressions to know which ones to get treated and which ones to leave alone.

I've seen when treatments are performed well, and it improves relationships with others but, most importantly, the relationship with self. When we know our best facial feature is being enhanced, we can feel comfortable in our skin.

> From the clinician's perspective, it's hard to get a great result if the Unique Facial Feature isn't being respected.

It takes time and expertise to examine each patient's face and personality and create a treatment plan that suits them uniquely. It requires creativity and dedication and a love of people that is not the glitz and glamour many new injectors dream it to be.

On the other hand, it's so easy to create a PUF. To put the same amount of product in each person's face in exactly the same areas so we all look the same, we all lose our ability to connect. That is easy. It's like using the same recipe for every single cake you bake. It will ensure consistency, but not individuality, which is why all PUFs look the same. That's why cosmetic medicine has turned from a legitimate medical specialty into a business opportunity, where seemingly everyone wants a piece of the pie.

## Medicine or Business.

A small high street near where I live has seven cosmetic businesses competing for the same customer dollars. In the marketing, we have a clinician pointing out all the ways our face is ageing. Not only is it depressing, but it's hard to practice restraint when the promise of erasing it all is flouted in front of us. And now we can buy even more for less. More package deals. 1, 2, 3, 4mls of dermal filler teamed with Botox for our frown, forehead, crow's feet, and more, all tied together in a neat little present on special for this-week-only. The problem with this is no one is getting assessed individually.

I've seen thousands of patients who've gotten sucked into buying these package deals. They often find they're injected with Botox and dermal fillers in areas they either didn't need or where it has, unfortunately, changed their face altogether. These deals promote a large amount of medicine for a discounted price. They also encourage women to have treatments they don't need to qualify for the discounted price. Facebook and Instagram have prohibited the advertising of these multi-package deals. If the main social media platforms are concerned enough about the harmful effect package deals are having on women, that's saying something.

Let's consider Stella's FEMs again.

STELLA CONTINUED.

I first saw Stella three months after she'd had the treatment that she felt changed her smile. While her crow's feet still hadn't regained their full muscle strength back, I could see that her eyes when she smiled, were her Unique Facial Feature. While Stella

31

talked, I examined her face <u>and</u> her personality, carefully.

From a very young age, we learn subliminally what our unique character and facial features are.

My youngest daughter has always been wise beyond her years. Her wee face tells a thousand stories of years gone by, and she says and does things more akin to a delightful little old lady. We've regularly told her she's a little comedian, so she has learned that her unique gift is to entertain us with her cunning wit and cheeky smile.

My eldest daughter's sincere looking eyes go between appearing blue and green, and we comment on how interesting this is. Now she automatically asks us, "What colour are my eyes today?" I can guarantee that her Unique Facial Feature as she grows, will be her unusual eye colour.

Stella's personality was light and relaxed. I felt comfortable in her presence immediately. I explained to Stella that her Unique Facial Feature is her eyes, that her crow's feet add sparkle to her eyes. It didn't surprise me that because of her 'smile changing' she felt unhappy. I described how if we wipe out the parts of our face that support our Unique Facial Feature, we wipe out our unique facial feature too. In treating Stella's crow's feet, she'd lost the warmth and joy of her personality. This made perfect sense to Stella. It comforted her to learn that perhaps there wasn't anything seriously wrong with her mood. That her husband and those around her were merely concerned at seeing a different Stella to the one they knew and loved. They weren't pointing out a personality flaw.

Stella's frown lines were strong both at rest and when she frowned. With Stella's crow's feet erased, her frown would've been more prominent, and her smile non-existent. No smile and a big frown would justify anyone to ask, "Stella, are you ok?"

The treatment we decided on was a non-treatment. We would not treat Stella's crow's feet with Botox as we didn't want to remove her ability to create her beautiful smile. We softened her frown lines and supported her lower crow's feet with dermal filler so that the crow's feet muscle could work at its best.

The result was lovely. At Stella's two-week review, she reported her crow's feet were finally returning to normal after the treatment 4 months ago. She was feeling more herself and smiling again. People asked her why she was so happy all the time. And guess what, the more people who told her she looked happy, the happier she felt.

---

Lesson:

Everyone's recipe should be different. It all depends on your unique facial feature and your unique personality feature. Keep the focus always on you. Never be swayed into doing what others do, they are not you, and you are not them.

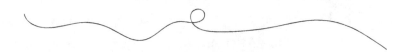

# Part Two

# APPEARANCES CAN BE DECEIVING.

## CASE STUDY: FIONA

I first saw Fiona in my waiting room five years ago, her face overfilled to the point of looking alien-like. Her cheeks were abnormally large and sharp, her eyes disappeared into her head and were almost hidden from too much tear trough dermal filler. In a heartbeat, I made a judgement that I'm not proud of, and worse still, was incorrect. I judged that Fiona was a 'shopper.' A 'shopper' is a term we use in the profession to refer to patients who go from clinic to clinic to get the lowest price. They often only come to a new clinic when disillusioned and angry that they can't have their unrealistic expectations met by their previous practitioner. Or their former practitioner has refused to treat them anymore.

When I saw Fiona, I immediately made a judgement in my head. I had my defences up and decided exactly how I would handle the situation. After treating many patients, clinicians get handy at recognising those whose behaviour elicits a 'red flag.' Unrealistic expectations, lack of acceptance over what is achievable for their face, and a refusal to listen to expert reason will all mean a 'red flag.' I gave Fiona a 'red flag' based on her looks.

*Fiona didn't meet my eyes as she asked, "Can you help me?"*

*"How can I help you?" I replied.*

*"Can you fix my face?"*

A common misconception that Body Dysmorphic shoppers have is that there's something innately wrong with their face.

*"Have you ever had treatment before?" I asked.*

Sometimes patients lie on their questionnaire to hide how many treatments they've had. It's like people who shop from GP to GP for opiate pain killers. They often say they haven't taken opiates before.

*"Twelve months ago, I had a treatment done by someone my friends recommended in the city. It was my first time." Fiona started to cry.*

*"What did you have done?" I asked.*

*"I had dermal fillers in my cheeks, and it made me look like this," Fiona whispered.*

*The penny dropped. Fiona wasn't a 'shopper' at all, but a patient who, against her will, had been over-treated. I'm seeing an alarming rate of these patients in my clinic.*

*Fiona continued, "I looked in the mirror after the doctor did the treatment. I was horrified. The doctor made me look like her. She thought I looked great, but I looked like her. I didn't think she looked great. She looked weird. Everyone who worked there looked the same."*

*Finally, Fiona looked me in the eyes for the first time.*

"*My face has been like this for twelve months now. It's ruined my life.*"

"*Did you go back to see the doctor?*" I enquired.

"*I called the clinic after a few days and was told I'd get used to how it looked and not to worry. They said it might just be swelling, and it can take time for the swelling to go down. After two weeks, I called again and said I didn't like the way it looked. But they wouldn't book another appointment for me to see the doctor for three months. I called again the following week, and they told me the doctor wasn't able to see me again.*"

## "It ruined my life."

*Fiona told me about the impact it had on her life. Since the dermal filler treatment to her cheeks, she'd become a hermit and refused to leave her house. Her husband told her she looked weird and wasn't sensitive to the impact it placed on her feelings of self-worth. She stopped socialising with family. She dropped out of her weekly catch up with her girlfriends, especially the ones who'd recommended Fiona have the treatment. In front of me sat a forty-five-year-old woman whose life was negatively impacted thanks to following a trend and being over-treated.*

"*I'm so depressed. I haven't looked in a mirror for almost a year. There's no way I can hide this with makeup. Wherever I go, everyone looks at me as if I'm weird, and I know people are talking about me behind my back.*"

*I comforted Fiona while she spoke. It was apparent she hadn't told anyone else this information before.*

"*I swore I'd never go near a place like this again, but I've been watching you in the local magazine. I've watched some of the women leave, and they all looked normal. And you look normal.*"

*"You are safe here, Fiona." I said.*

*"Can you fix my face?" Fiona asked.*

## Four dangers of becoming a Pretty Ugly Face.

**1. Pretty Ugly Faces don't look like themselves; they look like everyone else.**

It's what's most heartbreaking. Identical lips, cheeks, chins, jawlines, noses, frowns, foreheads, and crow's feet make it hard to identify the differences among women today.

Think about most reality TV shows. The women on TV who've had 'too much' treatment, look the same. It can be hard to differentiate. If you were to describe one by saying, "You know, the one with the big lips…" well, that might depict all of them. The one who can't talk properly because her 'lips are too big,' again, might describe them all.

Whenever a new reality TV show airs, I have an influx of patients who suddenly want to discuss the overdone faces on their TV screens. People ask my advice on 'why' the women have done this to themselves. It frightens and unsettles people. They're scared that it's the way they'll be expected to look too.

---

I recall a situation whereby a patient was trying to describe a reality TV star to me; *"You know the one, huge lips, can't speak properly, big eyelashes, hair extensions, puffy cheeks, always looks miserable, never smiles." I didn't watch the TV show, so I had no idea who it was, so we asked my skin therapist who stated, "You could be describing any of them."*

---

We only have a handful of facial features with which to differentiate ourselves from the next person. When those facial features are blown up, look out of proportion on our face, and look identical to every other over-treated woman, I believe people lose respect for us. People assume we're a bit of a joke, the jester, the fool, the villain. That we deserve to be made fun of and taunted. They assume that we have such poor self-control we deserve to be mocked and teased. The social opinion of us is low.

I can't exactly explain why this happens, but I've seen it in full effect.

Overdone faces also have a hard time proving to people that they are smart, sensitive, and strong women. They start from the back and often, regardless of their accomplishments and achievements, or how loud they yell, they are never judged relatively on their talents.

This brings us to the next concern I have. I hate to think of the objectification of these women. It's hard enough being on a reality TV show without having your looks scrutinised too. And all because you wanted to look your best, so you had the lips, cheeks, and Botox overdone. I discuss the pressure celebrities face in Chapter Nine. Because I believe there's a trick that we're all missing, it has perpetuated the problem we see with PUFs. Our inability to have faith in our Unique Facial Feature has led to the loss of our beauty.

## 2. Pretty Ugly Faces are less attractive than they were. They lose what makes them beautiful.

We've described when you dilute your Unique Facial Feature by enhancing another feature on your face; you lose the best part of your face. The part that makes you unique and beautiful.

In today's day and age, when we can pretty much have anything we want, it's tempting to have it all. I promise that once you know what your Unique Facial Feature is, you'll be empowered. You'll ignore the temptation to have treatments that aren't suitable for you and your Beautiful Unique Face.

If you have incredible, beautifully long legs, why on earth would you wear a sack over them permanently? When someone says, "You have wrinkles around your eyes, you need to get rid of those," that might be true for them. But for someone like Stella, it wasn't correct for her, and it might not be for you either.

## 3. Because of a lack of emotion, Pretty Ugly Faces look angry, unhappy, or pretentious.

We saw how with Stella, after she'd received too much Botox in her crow's feet, the muscle that pulled up her cheeks when she smiled became paralysed. It created a chipmunk-like appearance we've all seen before. As a quick reference, think of the negative media reports about Courteney Cox or Bethenny Frankel, after their initial forays into Botox.

Pretty Ugly Faces by nature have too much done to their faces and lose the ability to express any emotions, including happiness and joy. We just end up looking angry, bitter, and sad. A lack of emotion doesn't create a beautiful face. A lack of emotion creates a cold and indifferent demeanour. The person with this face always looks unapproachable, arrogant, and condescending. People tread carefully near them; they avoid them; they fear them, and so over-treated people often behave in a way that confirms these opinions.

We're all typecast based on our looks. Our behaviour mimics our appearance. Sincere and open impression? People will tell you all. Happy and cute face? People will expect you to cheer them up. Wise and experienced look? People will expect you to solve their problems. Frozen and emotionless face? People will treat you cautiously.

In turn, our appearance informs our personality. An over-frozen and overfilled face means we find it hard to meet people and create relationships based on first impressions. The reality is, most people who look like this are awesome women, and when you get to know them, they are warm and funny. So why do they want to look unapproachable?

For some, it's because they are trying to eradicate any signs of facial ageing or perceived imperfections. They aim to chase every single line and wrinkle off their face. It then becomes a way of life, a pattern that results in a habit. A face devoid of facial expressions looks the same when either happy or sad. Everyone thought Stella was unhappy when she wasn't. In turn, this led to Stella feeling unhappy. The power of suggestion from those around her made Stella think herself into a way of feeling.

**4. Pretty Ugly Faces look older than their actual age.**

On reality TV and social media, we're seeing young women in their 20s and early 30s, who no longer look like young women. They've had the nuances of their youthful faces erased. Much to their shock, it doesn't make them more attractive, it makes them less beautiful. It's paramount we get this message through to young women today. And it is equally important young men understand this, too. It's all of our responsibility to remove the expectation that this is how young women should look.

At my niece's 21st birthday party, I had a wonderful time looking at all the young women's faces. I worked out exactly why PUFs look older than they are.

When we're in our 20s, our skin bounces back after we express emotion. We frown, but as soon as we stop frowning, our skin becomes smooth and flat again. We smile, and our eyes crinkle as they should, yet as soon as we stop smiling, the skin around our eyes smooths out and relaxes.

Our skin's ability to return to smoothness after we have expressed the emotion is what gives our age away.

When we're young, our skin is plumper, and the lines are not as etched as when we're older. I describe it to my patients as a piece of paper of varying thicknesses. When we're younger, our skin is like thick, plump, moist, felt-like cardboard. It creates the muscle movement the emotion requires; smile, frown, worry, and so on, and then it bounces back. Because of the thickness of the paper, young people's skin doesn't entirely create the full depth of frown we create when we're older. But we know the emotion they express. There's no confusion about how a young person is feeling.

When older, our skin resembles thinner paper. When we create the emotion, not only does it look like we're expressing it more strongly, but it also stays in that emotion for longer. Sometimes because of the repetitive movement, just like the continuous folding of a piece of paper, we get a permanent line in the skin. It means the line is there when we aren't expressing the emotion, which is often misinterpreted as a mood.

When young women get too much injected into their faces, they lose the ability to express emotions. They also lose the marker that tells us how plump and youthful their skin is by bouncing back after expressing the emotion. It's why, when young women get too much done to their faces, they look older.

## Only older women get Botox and dermal fillers.

The next reason PUFs look older than their age is the assumption that only older women get injections into their faces. When a younger woman has an over-frozen and overfilled face, we assume she must be older. And not just a bit older than they are, but much older than their actual age. I have spoken to young women who have had too much treatment done, and people regularly think they're in their 40s. For a twenty-five-year-old woman, this is quite upsetting. And it is equally upsetting for the forty-year-old woman who ends up looking sixty. In my experience, it is only women in their 80s who benefit from having too much done. They look like they are in their 60s.

I have never had one patient ask me to make them look older than they are. Most of my patients don't even want to look drastically younger. But they do all want to look fresher and happier. More suitable and smaller treatments with expert clinicians will mean you can have the best of this and look your age but fresher and happier and never older. So, the advertisements for Botox that make the appeal about wiping out all your lines and wrinkles is totally wrong. It won't make you look younger; it will do the exact opposite.

Within that first appointment, Fiona was open and honest about her awful experience. I'd judged her as had others who'd come into contact with her after her initial treatment. I saw her overdone, overfilled, and strange-looking face and made a poor judgement on the state of her personality. Fiona lived her torture for twelve months. She'd received a look she didn't want, and she didn't request. It impacted her mental health and her happiness.

> Having injectable cosmetic treatments is not something to be considered lightly.
> It looks like every person has something or other done to their faces on social media, in the media or your social circle. That doesn't mean it's right for you, or that the treatment they've had is the best treatment for you.

FIONA CONTINUED.

It's challenging to make a 'best plan' when someone has had various treatments previous to seeing me. It's akin to asking an artist to paint over someone else's half-completed artwork. It's impossible to know the surface you're expected to build upon and make lovely, let alone what materials they have used.

Without knowing what Fiona looked like without dermal filler in her cheeks, it was challenging. I examined her face, but it was necessary not to assume anything. I went on what Fiona told me they'd treated her with, but I didn't know any of this to be fact. I could only rely on was what I saw with my own eyes, what I was feeling by palpating her face, and what happened to her face after I used a drug designed to dissolve the dermal filler used twelve months previously. I didn't know what type of dermal filler she'd received, and I wasn't sure if I could dissolve it with my dissolving medicine.

My initial assessment of Fiona was skewed based on her appearance as she sat in front of me.

I concluded that Fiona naturally had:
**1**. Prominent cheeks and tear troughs.
**2**. Small eyes in proportion to her face.
**3**. Hollow temples which contributed to the appearance of large cheeks.

Therefore, her Unique Facial Feature was her cheeks as they were the most prominent feature on her face.

We can actually create a Unique Facial Feature in someone's face through plastic surgery and cosmetic injectables. But this will <u>always</u> be to the detriment of their natural Unique Facial Feature. It's why inexperienced practitioners find it hard to assess individual faces and will treat only the wrinkles they see. A limited understanding of aesthetics or human psychology sees them only skilled on a basic level to create cheeks en masse, eyes en masse, lips en masse, and so on. They're building a sea of clones. It's more challenging to be skilled and practice restraint than to be haphazard and practice recklessly.

Fiona felt helpless. The impact the treatment placed on her life was detrimental.

I dissolved the dermal filler in Fiona's cheeks with a dissolving agent which works quickly. I could see within a few minutes of injecting it that her cheeks and the puffy under-eye area softened and reduced in size. It takes two weeks for it to fully dissolve and for any swelling or bruising from this treatment to settle.

I saw Fiona two weeks later and could now see her natural, unaltered face. Fiona told me that straight after her last appointment, she stopped into a cafe and enjoyed a coffee and a piece of cake. It was the first time she'd done that in twelve months. It was a huge breakthrough and signalled a return to a feeling of safety and normality that Fiona missed for a year.

The original assessment I made of Fiona's temple hollowing was still apparent, even with her cheek size significantly reduced. Still, it was nowhere near as dramatic as two weeks earlier. The effect of her overfilled cheeks made other areas of her face look abnormal. So, while she had a reasonable amount of temple hollowing, her overfilled cheeks and under-eye hollows made her look like she had an excessive amount of hollowing. If I'd filled these without first seeing what she looked like with no previous treatments, I would've always been playing catch-up and conceal.

Like the pimple you pick, then try to cover with makeup and concealer. It then gets infected and more substantial, creating more to cover up and irritating the infected pimple even more. Or the wall that collapses so you prop it back up with a dodgy repair. It is crucial to address the root issue first and then reassess.

If you can get things back to basics, creating a raw and neutral place to start, then it's ideal. We decided to add some dermal fillers in Fiona's temples. It dramatically helped to rebalance her face and soften the effects of ageing, which is what Fiona sought treatment for in the first place.

We started Fiona on prescribed topical creams for her skin and did a small amount of lower face Botox.

## You are unique. No one else is like you.

I've been treating Fiona for five years now and only twice a year. We've NEVER done any dermal fillers anywhere near her cheeks or under-eye hollows. Just because your friend, or the influencer on social media, or a clinician tells you they have this area treated does NOT mean you should have it done, too.

Your practitioner should only assess what **your** face needs and what's best for **you** and **your** personality, not what they've treated the last ten people with.

Five years on Fiona has more balanced facial proportions. A Unique Facial Feature that stands out for the right reasons. Beautiful eyes, highlighted by active and high crow's feet, which add sparkle and shine. Her eyes were hidden in our first consultation by her puffy cheeks and overfilled under-eye hollows. Now her face looks younger, happier and more refreshed. In her appointments, Fiona has a more positive mood - she regularly smiles, laughs and freely discusses her family, friends and home in a positive light.

The impact of a revised treatment plan with Fiona's Unique Facial Feature at the forefront has been positive, too.

Fiona reports being happier with her appearance than she has ever felt.

She has realistic expectations about what treatment is suitable for her and makes decisions based on all the information.

Fiona has realistic exceptions of ageing in her face and skin and knows what she can do to look her best.

Fiona is happy to take control of her feelings of worth based on her appearance.

Sadly, Fiona was unwittingly turned into someone else's idea of beauty and, when she didn't like it, she was ignored. Fiona didn't want it all. She wanted none of it.

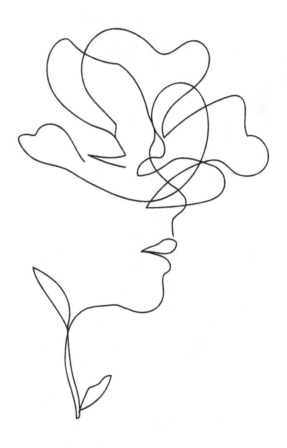

# Chapter Two

## Part One

# SEE IT, WANT IT, BUY IT, HAVE IT!

CASE STUDY: LUCY

### "I want it all now!"

Lucy was thirty years old when she first came to my clinic on a recommendation from a friend of hers. She attended her first appointment with her older sister.

With what I know about Lucy now, five years on, I should've refused to treat her at that very first appointment. If I had, I wouldn't have had years of turmoil and heartache trying to deal with her narcissistic personality.

Thankfully, in my years of practice, I've only come across two narcissistic patients. Interestingly, they're almost identical in looks, age, and behaviour. Up to where I felt brave enough to stand up to them, both managed to eat me alive.

I quickly learned Lucy was anorexic and body dysmorphic. She was preoccupied with cooking and counting calories. Lucy had an obsession with exercise to the point of exercising even when severely injured. She wore her anorexia and exercise addictions as badges of honour: Proud to tell others how little she'd eaten and how much exercise she'd done that day.

Lucy had very little to no affect. In the years she was my patient, I never saw her laugh or smile. She had a very skewed perception of herself, her personality, and her behaviour towards others. At the time of writing this book, it's been almost two years since seeing or speaking with Lucy. I seriously debated whether to put her in my book as the thought of her still causes me panic.

At the time of writing this book, I believe Lucy had a narcissistic personality disorder. She was probably also suffering the effects of chronic stress and the modern phenomena of needing to be perfect and have everything 'look just right'. She was likely obsessive compulsive and addicted to adrenaline and cortisol. I discuss this more in Chapter Ten but let me share Lucy's story first.

## Ageing isn't a race you can win.

Lucy obsessed over online shopping. She wore teeny tiny outfits that showed as much of her body as was legal. How thin she looked, how perfect her appearance and how well-fitting her outfit were, occupied the hours it took her to get ready to leave the house. Even a simple outing to the grocery store became an event. Lucy also thrived on competition. She would stay longer at work to produce better presentations than her colleagues. If Lucy saw someone thinner than her, she'd spiral into a manic phase of cooking, but not eating. If she saw someone with bigger cheeks or lips, or longer lashes or smoother skin, she'd up the ante and demand to have hers bigger/longer/smoother, too.

As Lucy grew older, beating ageing became another obsession. In her mind, I was the key to her beating ageing to a pulp and winning the race. Ageing is not a race that can be won, and she took it out on me with each loss she sustained. This story is not unique to me. I know many practitioners who've endured similar experiences.

Lucy always overstepped the mark in terms of professional boundaries. Constantly arguing over price and attempting to confuse staff and catch them out so she could pay less. Lucy insisted on eating into another patient's appointment time. Even when her allocated appointment time had been discussed and agreed, she'd claim she was being mistreated and made a song and dance. Lucy learned if she could book in at the very end of the day, she could force us to stay back later as we had no further patients waiting.

In addition to a love of winning and being right, Lucy's favourite thing to do was to bargain with my staff and me at every opportunity. Lucy regularly threatened to take her business elsewhere, sharing that she'd driven thirty minutes to see me. Patients regularly drive up to seven hours to see me and others even arrange their flights to Australia based on their next appointment with me. I would think that over 50% of the patients I see each day, drive one or more hours to see me, so Lucy's threat fell on deaf ears. I offered on many occasions to recommend a clinic closer to Lucy to attend, but she refused each time. I guess she enjoyed having that card up her sleeve.

## "I want to look completely flawless and perfect."

*At her very first appointment, Lucy said, "My lips are small. I want them to be bigger."*

*"I would like to examine your face if that's ok and suggest what treatment is best for you based on your Unique Facial Feature," I said.*

*"I want to look completely flawless and perfect," Lucy replied.*

*"How do you mean?" I questioned.*

*"I've seen these girls"- points to her phone - "I want you to make me look like that. I know what they've had done to their faces."*

*The girls on the phone were not "real" in that their faces were heavily filtered and photoshopped versions of how they really looked.*

*"How do you know what treatments they've had done?" I asked.*

*"It says it here in the comments, look."*

*Indeed, the comment stated the filtered faces I was looking at each had a 'little sprinkling of anti-wrinkle around the eyes, frown and forehead, a little touch of dermal filler to their lips and cheeks for a very natural-looking result.'*

*I almost gagged. There was nothing natural-looking about the faces on the phone. It gave me a good insight into what brainwashed Lucy.*

*"I want to have my Botox here, here, here and here," she said, pointing to every area of her face. "I want fillers in my lips, my cheeks and under my eyes and I read that you can do dermal fillers in the nose, I want that too. I also want the Kim Kardashian vampire treatment on my skin."*

*I explained to Lucy that given this was the first time she'd had treatment, we'd decide together what was best for her face, based on her one Unique Facial Feature. We'd then break her treatment plan into different treatment sessions.*

*"Oh no, I don't want only one unique feature. I want all my features to be unique, and I want it all done now," she said.*

This last statement pretty much sums up the mindset of people like Lucy. They don't appreciate the subtle nuances of a beautiful face, **wanting it all and wanting it now**.

## The PUFs are taking over.

Everywhere I look, their Pretty Ugly Faces are staring expressionless back at me. Filled to the brim with dermal fillers and Botox, I'm unsure where to look. There is no escape from them. On my Instagram feed, in my local cafe, at the train station, and in the hundreds, PUFs are in my clinic waiting room.

The PUF experience isn't isolated to women in their 40s, 50s, or 60s. I see women from eighteen to eighty suffering from the PUF epidemic.

What the hell have we created? And how do we find our way back to our unique beauty?

I believe we look to people who are 1-2 steps ahead in life to guide, inspire, and lead us. In the modern world, this means we look to people with more celebrity, success, and wealth than us. We aspire to be, do, and have what they have.

Today, every street corner has a franchise clinic offering to eradicate your frown, fill up your cheeks, and give you the perfect chiselled jaw. They'll plump up your lips like whichever Kardashian sister is posting and pouting most on her Instagram account.

You can see how we are in the grip of a PUF epidemic. Despite what the girls and women lining up for their syringe-fix think, it's not making anyone pretty. It's turning us all into cyborg-like clones and a dangerous sea of Pretty Ugly Faces.

## See it, want it, buy it, have it.

This is our life motto. We live in a quick-fix society. We rely on instant gratification to give us hits of serotonin and endorphins for pleasure. Often, we get these from peer acceptance via social media posts and, dare I say it, quick-fix cosmetic injectables.

We live in a community that struggles with a lack of meaningful connection despite being 'connected' and visible 24/7. The subsequent isolation, anxiety, and the expectations we place on ourselves to be prettier, thinner, fitter, happier, and more successful than ever is real. It makes it easy to see why our human need to belong is often met with hits of social media consumption.

## The 'influencer' curse.

Social media shows us the glamorous lives of heavily filtered and edited influencers. They are the 'picture perfects' who, I'll continue to remind you, are paid enormous amounts of money for endorsements. They're literally paid to tell you about how happy a product or service has made them, even if it is a lie. In a nutshell, our modern-day marketing consists of approaching an 'influencer' who has a decent following on their social media page, made up of possible customers who are likely to not only be sucked into believing any shiny-happy-story but furthermore, buy the product being endorsed by the influencer.

As a cosmetic enhancement clinician with a busy clinic, and a social media presence, I'm approached daily. Not only by influencers themselves but by their agents who flatter me by telling me they identified me as a high-profile business. They say that, with the help of an influencer, I can increase my customer base and dollar turnover.

A recent email made my stomach turn:

*'We handle the whole process from recruiting the best-suited influencers (young women in their 20s are proving best for your industry) to driving thousands to your site and clinic, so you can sit back and watch the $$ pour in...'*

I'm a practitioner in a medical clinic, prescribing and administering schedule 4 pharmaceutical drugs. They want me to give a treatment to a young woman who can then publish a gushing post about how amazing it is, how it's improved her life and made her happier. They're asking me to exacerbate a society in crisis. They encourage me to increase the promotion and usage of highly controlled medicines in women who are already vulnerable, confused, but, most importantly, don't require the drug. Their attempt to lure me in with the promise of increasing the money I can make is not only medically unsafe, but also unethical and immoral. But it's happening. And there are plenty of clinics who are grasping the opportunity, regardless of the cost to women and their physical or mental health.

Many things strike me when I receive these requests. First, it is illegal to give away scheduled medicine for the promise of a shout out. Second, the influencers they are parading in front of me like some sick beauty contest DO NOT NEED COSMETIC INJECTABLES. Third, the people following their influencer's page are being lied to by the marketing agent and the influencer.

Despite what the photos supposedly show, the influencers are *not* the happiest they have ever been, with their Pretty Ugly Faces. Their overfilled lips have *not* made them the best person they have ever been. They are *not* winning, living their very best lives, and filling their cup of love to the brim because of their newly chiselled jaw.

Truth be known, many of these influencers (who I've treated as private patients) are on a multitude of anti-anxiety and antidepressant medications. They're usually riddled with self-doubt, crippled by a lack of self-worth, and they hate their PUFs. Their golden handcuffs keep them in the role of influencer because of the money they know they can earn. And, because they are often young women, they feel their looks, bodies, and overall appeal to an audience is the only way they can earn money.

Out of the spotlight the influencers I've met pay the price from the extreme pressure of always being 'on.' Their mental and physical health suffers because they are continuously swallowing down the pretence of perfection. More than most, they are expected to put on the happy face and sell the lie that the product/service/cosmetic injectable treatment is responsible for the joy they show in their post.

## Is it medicine or is it business?

In Australia, we are seeing the use of Botox and dermal filler injections rising faster than ever before. We estimate that Australia's cosmetic procedure business is about $1bn, which is 40% larger per capita than the United States. But what is often seen and promoted as a low-risk procedure is not akin to having your eyebrows waxed or haircut. Botox and dermal fillers are far from risk-free.

## Last year in Australia, we had the first case of blindness from dermal fillers.

According to reports, the patient may not have been warned about the potential for blindness. She started complaining about vision loss during the procedure. Still, the practitioner performing the treatment didn't administer the dissolving agent that could've potentially saved her vision.

The ophthalmology department treated the woman as a medical emergency in Sydney's Prince of Wales Hospital, but they couldn't save her vision. It seems the practitioner injected the dermal filler into an artery, which directly supplies blood to the eye. Once the dermal filler blocks the artery, the eye slowly dies, resulting in blindness.

Meanwhile, in Asia, a thirteen-year-old girl convinced a clinic she was over eighteen, and they didn't request identification. The young girl is now permanently blind in one eye, thanks to having dermal filler injected into her nose. Her parents thought she was at a friend's house listening to music.

---

**How I recognise (and how you can avoid becoming) a Pretty Ugly Face:**
**1.** Lips are huge and out of proportion for their face.
**2.** Inability to speak properly because of overfilled lips *and or* an over-relaxed mouth muscle.

---

**3.** Cheeks that are so puffy they sit too high and obliterate and push up the lower eyelid, making their eyes appear smaller. *And / or* cheeks that are over defined and sharp that their face looks almost alien-like.

**4.** An obsession with every line and wrinkle on their face.

**5.** A feeling of overwhelm and panic at the appearance of a line or wrinkle on their face. Leading to attempting everything hoping to erase all lines and wrinkles. Babies and small children naturally have small lines and wrinkles on their faces. It's ok.

**6.** A feeling of overwhelm and panic that their face (lips, cheeks, jawline) is deflating like a punctured tyre and needs to be filled up urgently.

**7.** A puffy, pillowy, blown up face.

**8.** An obsession with the social media accounts of Cosmetic Medicine clinics and clinicians who produce Pretty Ugly Faces.

**9.** An obsession with the social media accounts of influencers who regularly gushingly post about their injectable treatments.

**10.** A fixation that injectables will make them happy and obsessing over the next part of their face that needs 'fixing.'

**11.** Ridiculously unrealistic expectations of their face and, therefore, their cosmetic clinician who they believe has the power to erase all lines and wrinkles magically.

**12.** The use of a face-changing app and filter to make them appear 'more attractive,' 'younger,' 'glamorous,' 'celebrity,' and so on.

**13.** An inability to see when someone has had too much dermal filler or Botox injected.

With practitioners vying for business on social media with hashtags like #mypatientsarehotterthanyours posted alongside the image of a twenty-something-year-old woman wearing next to nothing, it's no wonder we are a society in crisis. I can't imagine Paediatricians posting pictures of ill children promoting #mypatientsaresickerthanyours to build their business. It's a disgusting abuse of power.

Current affairs, media outlets, and cosmetic medicine associations are doing their best to expose a growing concern and educate the public. Still, the horse has already well and truly bolted. And those of us trying to pull on its reins are failing miserably at upholding standards of ethical practice.

## From two hours to four days to become an 'expert'.

Private training companies and now even plastic surgeons are jumping on the lucrative bandwagon of growth. They charge anywhere between $5,000 - $20,000 for courses aimed at GPs, Nurses, and Dentists. These courses range from two hours to four days, with a significant component being online rather than in person. Most training companies are also creating buying groups. This way, their students get the promise of ongoing discounted product so they can start treating the public the same day they finish their short course. It's often from an unregistered setting, or in a Botox party environment a patient's house (which is highly illegal).

From a clinical perspective, it is effortless to create a PUF. It's why anyone can open a clinic, lure vulnerable members of the public in, start filling them up, and churning them out. What is more complicated, however, is to skilfully treat a face to look aesthetically fresher, softer, happier, more beautiful, and, perhaps *most* importantly, normal. That ability takes an advanced artistic 'aesthetic eye', which is developed over many years and considers aspects of patient safety first and foremost.

I'm not saying you're not allowed to have anything done at all. I've performed thousands of treatments and own a bustling cosmetic medicine clinic, so that would be crazy, unrealistic, and, quite frankly, a ridiculous career move. No way! Why on earth? Are you kidding? It would be like asking you to throw away your smartphone. It's 2020. Cosmetic injectables are commonplace and considered standard maintenance, like going to the hairdresser.

The makers of Botox - Allergan, launched a marketing campaign trying to convince millennials to have Botox with their 'Are you bo-curious?' advert. **https://www.businessinsider.com.au/allergan-ad-campaigns-targeting-millennials-2018-9?r=US&IR=T    9/6/2020.**

Their business objective is to ensure everyone has injectables like they buy shampoo, so with marketing power (money) behind those who want you to have treatments, you've little hope of never having anything done. However, if you do it, you can move forward with a plan of what your Unique Facial Feature is and therefore have it done well.

## "I don't want too much." OR "I don't want it to be too noticeable."

Few of the over-treated women I've met started their journey into cosmetic injections with the dream of becoming over-treated. If anything, most begin their journey saying something like, "I don't want too much," or "I don't want it to be too noticeable." However, like all sneaky addictions, it can creep up and take over.

One minute we think we're nicely in control—just a bit here, a bit there. And the next minute we want more and more done, then bam—we're down that rabbit hole! Without realising, we have become over-treated. Without an idea of what our Unique Facial Feature is, this is more than likely to happen. That is why I am proud of the women I have treated. Whether they be first-timers or seasoned patients from elsewhere, once they know what their Unique Facial Feature is, they know how to ensure they honour their beautiful, unique face and never look over-treated.

I aim to teach you what I share with every one of my patients; how to stay safe and keep your wits about you in a world where, if you're not careful, you'll find yourself on that high-speed train heading for destination Pretty Ugly Face (PUF).

## The Good, The (Reformed) Bad and the Ugly

In this book, I share the stories of a variety of cosmetic medicine patients of mine who represent the *Good*, the *(Reformed) Bad*, and the *Ugly* in terms of how cosmetic medicine is playing out in the faces of society.

## Is it too late?

When I started working in this industry, I never imagined I would be in this position: A successful practitioner writing a book about how *not* to have treatments that change your face too much. Perhaps some people will assume I've become an anti-treatment advocate. But my motivation to get into this industry all those years ago on the film set has intensified as the access to, and obsession with, cosmetic injectables has taken on a life of its own. Not only are we paralysing our muscles, we're deadening our ability to see what faces us in the mirror. If we take action now, recognising that Botox and fillers *can* be used, but with care instead of impulse, then perhaps all is not lost.

Our minds are like sponges. All the messages and stimuli we get today through social media activates our Fear of Missing Out (FOMO). We doubt that we are pretty enough, thin enough, fit enough, strong enough, successful enough, rich enough, entrepreneurial enough, just...enough. We are continually sold things in a way that negatively sparks our attention.

Fear is an excellent way to get our attention. It makes us take action. By telling us that the only way we can be happy is by having the stuff that's for sale, is a sure method to buy. The intention behind every post is to cause an emotional reaction within us so we feel inadequate and buy into the belief that whatever they're selling, we need. Now that every person can sell to us via their own private

Instagram page, we're bombarded by the messages telling us we're inadequate.

## Having a social media account doesn't give you the right to be cruel. Stop it now!!

I've also noticed some of these people's behaviour is downright cruel, and I'm not surprised that online bullying is at an all-time high. I watched, with disbelief, the Instagram story of a former reality TV star turned influencer. Horrified to see the way she spoke to her mother and her partner in the livestream. Nasty words, swearing, name calling, mockery and bullying. Calling her mother stupid and her partner ugly. Saying to her mother, "You're so annoying, I wish I wasn't your daughter," and to her partner, "You're a waste of space, I deserve someone better," is not entertainment, it's glamorising bullying. Instagram stories give the illusion of reality TV.

> At a time when kindness is the only thing we need in the world today, watching people who are influencing our youth and us treat the people in their lives so poorly in the name of entertainment, is utterly disgraceful.

LUCY CONTINUED.

Lucy came to that first appointment with her sister. They hadn't made an appointment for her sister so the allocated time for Lucy had to be split consulting her and her sister. And treating them both. It was obvious at that point that I needed to take control of the situation, yet I didn't.

*"My sister is a mess; you need to fix her,"* Lucy stated.

*Her sister wasn't 'a mess.' She was an elegant woman in her mid-40s.*

*"I think your sister is lovely,"* I replied.

*"My sister needs the whole works, but she probably can't afford it, she doesn't have a job. She needs to be told what to do. I'll help her decide what she needs."* Lucy said.

*Lucy's sister smiled at me shyly. Maybe she was embarrassed, too. I certainly was. Lucy wasn't though. She was serious. It gave me an insight into what Lucy thought was an appropriate manner to speak to others.*

Over time, Lucy added to her list of obsessions, researching which treatments she could request. I noticed her addiction to exercise grew, and her anorexia seemed to worsen. She would attend each appointment with a photo of what she wanted to look like by the end of it.

## "All of my friends behave like this."

In the weeks and days leading up to her appointment, Lucy would call and text to ensure we knew what she was expecting from us. I thought of ways to discuss her declining mental health with her. At her next appointment with me, I broached the subject with Lucy.

*"Lucy, do you spend a lot of time looking at yourself in the mirror and considering things wrong with your face and body?"*

*"Yes, but that's because there are things wrong with my face."* Quickly, Lucy clocked on. *"I'm not body dysmorphic if that's what you're trying to imply."*

*It took me aback, but it wasn't altogether surprising that Lucy knew where my line of questioning was going.*

*"Do you feel it would help to talk to someone about the*

*expectations you have on yourself?"*

*"No. All of my friends behave like this."*

*And with that, the door was closed, and Lucy wouldn't hear another word of it.*

On one occasion, I told Lucy I wouldn't be able to treat her sister unless I could have a conversation with her without Lucy interjecting and speaking over her. I needed to gain informed consent from her sister and being coerced into having treatment by Lucy wasn't a way I could gain it. At one particular tense standoff between Lucy and her sister, I took a stand.

*"You need to have it done. You look so old," Lucy said, trying to convince her sister to have a thread lift.*

*"I don't know," her sister said. "It's more money than I can afford, and I don't know if I want anything more than a little Botox in my frown lines."*

*Lucy was growing angry. "You're so frustrating!"*

*"It needs to be your sister's choice, Lucy," I said.*

*"I've got to go to the toilet," Lucy said.*

*The minute Lucy left the room, I asked her sister what she'd like to do.*

*"I don't even want to be here," she said. "No offence to you, but I don't see why I need to have anything done."*

*With this information, I could be Lucy's sister's advocate. "Well, in that case, you should have nothing done. I will explain to Lucy that we've left it for now."*

*When Lucy returned, I told her that her sister and I had discussed all the treatment options and, for now, we would leave it. Lucy's sister smiled with thanks to me.*

Over the years of treating Lucy, despite being fairly experienced in my field, Lucy always wanted to know why I wasn't doing some treatment or other to her she'd seen on Instagram. She always wanted to know the in-depth details of every single treatment. Lucy needed to be told over and over what was best for her and why.

Lucy received skin peels, Botox, dermal fillers, skin needling, laser, and IV vitamin infusions from me over the years. By the end of our relationship together, she'd become uncontrollably demanding and histrionic in her behaviour.

## When your gut tells you to run a mile from someone, run a mile.

I feel like I did my absolute best with Lucy. Still, I should've asked her to seek treatment elsewhere, long before I did. Again, I felt a sense of responsibility to keep her from becoming a full blown PUF. With the body dysmorphia, anorexia and exercise addiction Lucy already had; she was a prime candidate for becoming a PUF. It was a constant battle with her to keep her mindset healthy. I failed her and she made my life hell. But, gee, she taught me a valuable lesson: When your gut tells you to run a mile from someone, run a mile.

In the lead up to my asking Lucy to seek treatment elsewhere, her aggression and manipulation were unacceptable. I was relieved to close the door to Lucy after her last appointment. Lucy seeks treatment from various other practitioners now. Although she's continued to contact my clinic hoping to make an appointment and acquire medicines I prescribe, I have and will always refuse her. My job is not to save all the women especially when one, such as this one in particular, is unwilling to first save herself.

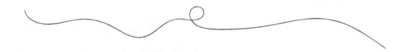

# Part Two

# "I'M OBSESSED WITH PHOTOS ON SOCIAL MEDIA."

CASE STUDY: NESSIE

Meet twenty-nine-year-old Nessie. Nessie had no idea what her Unique Facial Feature was. Still, by the time I'd met her, she'd already had a breast and nose augmentation as well as liposuction to her body.

Nessie contacted me at her grandmother's insistence after telling her she was going back to her plastic surgeon to have further liposuction and a facelift. Nessie's grandmother contacted me initially with her concern about her granddaughter's plans. I agreed to talk with Nessie before her planned surgery. I viewed a photo of Nessie before we chatted. The first thing I noticed was Nessie's stand out eyes.

Knowing Nessie's grandmother, I saw the similarities in their faces. I could anticipate how Nessie's face would change over time because of hereditary factors. I consulted Nessie over FaceTime so

I could hear her concerns firsthand and work out if there was a way to avoid going under the knife again. Following the consultation, Nessie agreed to postpone her surgery and see me.

*I initially saw Nessie in the waiting room of my clinic. Having only seen her in a photo and on FaceTime, I was pleased Nessie's eyes were far more unique than technology portrayed them.*

*Nessie was open and honest with me. We'd already shared a candid conversation during which Nessie told me she wanted bigger lips, the fat sucked out of her cheeks, liposuction under her chin, and the skin surgically pulled back with a facelift. She also wanted a stronger jawline.*

*"I'm obsessed with photos on social media," Nessie confided while in my treatment room.*

*Nessie was an intelligent, well-educated young woman. Employed in an incredible job, Nessie was witty and articulate. She'd also become addicted to looking at Instagram influencers.*

*"Even though I know they're not real, that's not what they look like in real life; I'm obsessed with these people on social media,"Nessie confessed.*

*Nessie showed me her phone. She had separate folders for each feature of her face and each area of her body. Within each folder, she had hundreds of photos she'd saved.*

'Lips.' 'Cheeks.' 'Jaw.' 'Mouth.' 'Neck.' 'Eyes'
'Forehead.' 'Hair.' 'Profile.' 'Breasts.' 'Arms.'
'Hands.' 'Fingers.' 'Stomach.' 'Thighs.' 'Butt.'
'Knees.' 'Calves.' 'Feet.' 'Toes.' 'Clothes.'
'Fitness.' 'Weight loss diets.' 'Food.' Nessie flicked through the photos from each of the folders for me.

What I saw was horrifying. An extensive catalogue of grotesque and overfilled lips, cheeks, and other facial features, body parts, and food plans impossible to strive for, let alone achieve, was a constant reminder to Nessie of how much she hated herself. The poor darling child. The PUFs were trying to suck Nessie down the rabbit hole. In one last-ditch effort to save herself, she'd bravely told her grandmother of her plans for more surgery, which led them both to me.

*"I want these lips and these cheeks, and the surgeon told me he could give me a jawline like this. He even said I would look so much prettier if I did..."*

*At this point, Nessie began to cry.*

*"I constantly look at myself in the mirror and compare myself to these women. I can't seem to help it. It's an addiction now."*

*"You think I am critical of my face. I'm worse with my body, but that's another story. My ex-husband commented about a woman's figure on Instagram once and asked me why my thighs didn't look like hers. I starved myself for days trying to change my body. To make my thighs look like hers. I got very sick. I ended up in the hospital for a week."*

*As she cried, I comforted her. I didn't speak, for I was so shocked that this genuinely stunning, kind, and bright young woman had been let down by so many people:*

*The surgeon who first operated on her at twenty-five years of age and then had subsequently agreed to do her second round of surgery in a few weeks. Which confirmed Nessie's belief that she wasn't enough and would be 'prettier' only once she'd had more surgery.*

*Her ex-husband for comparing her to another woman who wasn't even real.*

*Social media for lying to her and forcing her into such a whirlwind of self-loathing.*

*And, ultimately, the societal conditioning now considered standard for young women. Which places them under such incredible, terrible pressure to make drastic changes and continuously strive for an unrealistic beauty 'ideal.'*

*"Nessie, have you heard of body dysmorphia?" I asked.*

*"Yes, I have."*

*"Has anyone ever suggested you might have body dysmorphia?" I asked.*

*"No."*

*"Has anyone ever suggested you speak to someone about how you feel about your face and body? How you feel about yourself?" I asked.*

*"No, no one."*

Nessie was severely body dysmorphic. I knew it. Her surgeon would have known it. Her ex-husband would know it. The hospital where she was admitted following her attempt to achieve unachievable thighs knew it. Still, so far, no one had ever taken Nessie in hand and attempted to help her. I referred Nessie to a psychologist to get help with her mental health.

## Your Beautiful Unique Face.

Dear reader, what I explained to Nessie that day can help you, too.

*"Nessie, can you take this mirror, please?" I asked.*

*She did.*

*"Look at your face, and I will tell you what I see."*

*Nessie kept the mirror in her lap and shook her head.*

*"Look at your eyes for me. They're incredible. They are your Unique Facial Feature. Your eyes are beautiful."*

70

*Nessie lifted and looked into the mirror, "I can't see it," she said.*

*"Your face is perfectly designed to draw the focus back to your eyes. Your face is heart-shaped. The widest part of your face is the area from your cheekbones up to your eyebrows. It's where your large, perfectly shaped, and loving eyes are housed. Your lips, petite and placed like a little love heart, again draw the eye briefly down to your mouth, only to bounce our attention immediately back up to your eyes."*

*Nessie started to cry again.*

*"Nessie, look at your eyes. They're up there with the loveliest eyes I've ever seen, and I have seen a few pairs of eyes," I said.*

*Nessie stopped crying and was now looking at her eyes, really looking at her eyes. As if for the first time in her life.*

*I explained it to Nessie.*

*"Whatever we do to you, whatever you do in the future, you must always keep in mind that your eyes are your natural Unique Facial Feature. Like a piece of art where the summer garden is what the artist intends to be the main feature. If another artist came along and made the house more prominent and faded the garden into the background, your eye would no longer be attracted to the beautiful garden. It's the same with your face, Nessie. Your beautiful eyes are what you've been given as your standout Unique Facial Feature. If we play around with making your lips bigger, they'll become the focus of your face, and your eyes will lose their uniqueness. You can't fake what you've been given naturally, ever. Although women can chase Angelina's lips from a syringe, their lips will never look as real and beautiful as Angelina's lips. You can't beat nature at its own game."*

*"What about my moon face?" Nessie asked.*

*"Ok, so let's look at what is happening here. You have beautiful full cheeks. Your fat pads are young and wonderfully full. I create cheeks like these in people because not everyone is as blessed as you are to have them naturally. What we can do, with a tiny amount of dermal filler, is to create a slight sharpness to your cheeks so that again, ALL the attention is being pulled up to your eyes," I explained.*

*Nessie thought about this.*

*"You grind your teeth, yes?" I asked.*

*"All the time."*

*"Does the grinding give you headaches?" I asked.*

*"Yes, I wake with headaches."*

*"Cup your hands on your face like this, now clench your teeth. Can you feel your grinding muscles pop out when you do that?"*

*"Yeah, wow," Nessie said.*

*"We can reduce your headaches by weakening and slimming down the muscle responsible for your teeth grinding. This will reduce the roundness of your lower face," I said.*

*"Really? And it will help my headaches, too?"*

*"Absolutely. Remember, your eyes are your Unique Facial Feature. We need to do everything in our power to continue nature's work and make your eyes the prominent feature while making the other features of your face fade into the background," I explained.*

## Your Unique Facial Feature is your lead actor.

This resonated with Nessie, and she was becoming an active member of her treatment plan.

*I described it further. "We have lead actors and supporting actors for a reason. If all the actors in a film were lead actors, for one, there would be no story with nuances and pulls and pushes of character journeys. And, second, what a loud and ghastly film it would be! Every actor and character vying for the spotlight. As an audience, we'd lose interest and soon leave the theatre. Your facial features are no different."*

*"That makes sense." Nessie agreed.*

*"Your eyes are your lead actor. The rest of your features are in a supporting role and remain doing just that, supporting the lead actor. This way, we honour the truth of your facial story. What I don't want to do is make your jaw stronger or more prominent or your lips bigger. Everything we do will be to draw the audience's eye back to your lead actor, your eyes."*

*With genuine shock, Nessie commented, "I never knew my eyes were nice. Everyone has always called me 'moon face'."*

I performed the treatment I'd recommended. One millilitre of dermal filler to the sweet spot in Nessie's cheeks. It reduced any hint of roundness and made her full cheeks fade into the background which drew the attention back up to Nessie's eyes. A small amount of Botox in her teeth grinding muscles to stop her grinding and decrease the size of jaw muscles, complimented her sweetheart shaped face. Finally, some of my own medical grade skincare to minimise Nessie's acne flare-ups and reduce scarring.


NESSIE CONTINUED.

I saw Nessie two weeks later when her treatment had fully kicked in. She and I were delighted with her result and, while she had a long way to go and needed more help from her psychologist, she was well on the way to healing.

Identifying her UNIQUE FACIAL FEATURE was the first step in making Nessie take control of her life. Once she knew what was unique and special about her face, she could look at the pictures on Instagram and appreciate them for what they were: often heavily filtered and photoshopped pictures of other people different from her. They were not her.

> An even better plan was to mitigate Nessie's use of social media altogether, but this would take considerable effort.

Nessie told me, "It's weird. Since my treatment, everyone has commented about my eyes being beautiful. I'm not sure if it's because what you did has made my eyes stand out more or because now, I know that my eyes are my Unique Facial Feature. I am most happy with them."

*"I would say it's a combination of both," I offered.*

*"And to think, I was all ready to have surgery."*

*"You don't need surgery, Nessie. **You just needed to discover your Peeps.**"*

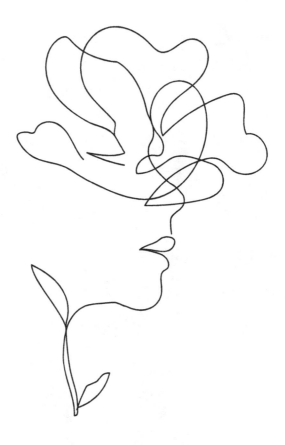

# Chapter Three

## Part One

## MEET YOUR PEEPS.

## Your Inner Power Practice will make you more beautiful.

Step 1. Peeps

Step 2. Tapping

Step 3. Mantra

### Step 1. Meet Your Peeps

You know that awful feeling you get when you ogle someone's social media page? In no time, intrigue turns into the familiar weight of overwhelm.

The more you pry into their life, the more it highlights your imperfections and shortcomings. Before you know it, you've not only lost a massive chunk of time that you could have better spent in other ways, but you've also lost a sense of self-love and worth.

# INNER POWER PRACTICE

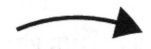

## PEEPS
- check in with them
- talk to the quiet ones
- ask them how they are, what they are feeling and then just sit and listen

## TAPPING
- on what your Peeps tell you
- see what comes up

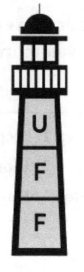

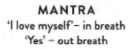

## MANTRA
'I love myself' – in breath
'Yes' – out breath

This feeling can become addictive, so before you know it, you're incapacitated yet cannot stop gawking at the pages of people who make you feel this way. Then you believe the only way you can feel happy is to emulate them. It might be a friend, a colleague, an influencer or a celebrity's page that you spend too much time ogling.

You wonder why you keep going back there. Why you keep teasing yourself with images that ultimately make you feel so awful. The behaviour becomes addictive because, each time you look at these images, your brain releases the neurotransmitter dopamine. Dopamine is our feel-good neurotransmitter. It reinforces and rewards behaviour that gives us pleasure.

## I'm addicted and so are you.

Just like the pleasure and satisfaction we get when eating a delicious piece of cake, we get the same hit when we look at images of 'beautiful people' on social media. So, what do we do to feel good? We keep going back for more. The quick hit we get outweighs the hours of self-loathing we may experience afterward. That is how powerful our brain chemicals are. We're geared for pleasure, seeking it out at every opportunity.

There are unscrupulous people out there in the world of social media and within cosmetic medicine clinics. They'll make you believe you need stuff you just don't need. They'll play on your insecurities. It's why we need an internal barometer to gauge what is right and what is terrible and guide us to make decisions that are best for us. I call this internal barometer, my Peeps.

## Let your Peeps guide you.

For nearly two decades now, I have called on my Peeps to guide me. Let me tell you who they are. Imagine you have one hundred little mini versions of yourself sitting (or hovering) in a big group inside your body. I feel mine around my solar plexus, and they all look like me. They are miniature versions of me and are all identical.

My Peeps primary function is to keep me safe. Collectively, they're my best friend and chief protector. If I feel uncertain about something, I ask my Peeps what they think and feel. I try to check in with my Peeps regularly too. I'll ask, "How are you feeling?" and I'll wait patiently for their answer. They might be silent for a few minutes while they consider the question or yell out a resounding solid answer. Some of your Peeps may answer, while others remain quiet. It's the quiet ones you want to explore further. Ask them what is going on with them? Ask them specifically how they feel? It may even be one Peep who is silent. Hone in on this one. Give it some attention and ask: "What's going on with you, little one?" Then wait patiently for their response. Like a litter of puppies, focus on each and then on the ones who are hiding behind the others.

Remember, they exist to keep you safe, not necessarily to keep you happy or always to experience that pleasure feeling I described earlier (aka, the dopamine hit.) Life isn't always just the highs. Waves have peaks and troughs, and so, too, does life. To expect to be happy ALL the time is setting yourself up for failure and disappointment. Be realistic and, if your Peeps or even one Peep, says they're not feeling so good, ask them to tell you what is going on. It'll be a concern you're already aware of, or it's something your subconscious is worrying about that you haven't yet consciously considered.

Your Peeps are your internal protectors. I find it is nice to check in with them when I'm feeling happy. Ask them, "Hey, are you guys ok?" Chances are they'll say, "Yeah, we're awesome," and even that bit of confirmation, for your happy mood, is like a mini celebration. A win for you and your team!

Sometimes you'll check in with your Peeps, and they will be seriously chilling out, and you disturbing them will kind of rouse them from a light slumber. But don't worry when this happens because it means they aren't worrying about anything. And then you, too, can breathe and let your worries go for now.

If you're feeling unsettled or anxious about something, but you can't quite put your finger on it, ask your Peeps to guide you. They will tell you precisely what is going on and why, and what they think you need to do about it. It might be merely to dedicate some thinking time to a particular person or thing. Either way, thank your Peeps for their care and do as they ask. Think about the person or something they have suggested and check in with them again once you have some clarity on the situation.

Your Peeps are your subconscious, and your subconscious is your guide. If we can open the channels for our subconscious to speak to us freely, we can solve many of the great mysteries of our own life.

## "When did you last check in with your Peeps, Anita?"

I told my husband about the conversations I had with my Peeps about sixteen years ago. He listened intently and, rather than thinking I was crazy, said how he liked my Peeps protecting me. Since that day, when I find myself in a psychological pickle (which happens more often than I'd like to admit), my husband asks me to check in with my Peeps and see how they're doing. By the time the psychological pickle has taken hold, it has often been months since I last checked in with my Peeps. So being reminded by my other biggest protector to check in with them, always works a treat.

I realise there's a direct correlation between how much I've neglected my Peeps and the depth of my psychological pickle. The longer it's been, the more likely it is that I find myself in a predicament. If I check in with them regularly, tend to them, keep our lines of communication open, and a pickle arises, it's often dealt with quickly and doesn't turn into a bigger problem. A near-miss, you might say.

Life is a wave, and while it's nice to ride the crest of the wave, it's equally as lovely to sit back and relax in the trough and regroup. Anything that we can do to avoid drowning every time that wave dips down is a win. Your Peeps will empower you to see the troughs as moments of contemplation and calm and just as important as the exciting highs of riding the crest.

Have you ever watched surfers just sitting on their boards, letting the swell of the waves take them up and down? If you're a surfer, you know how lovely it is to surrender. Let the ocean take you on its journey.

## Identifying your Beautiful Unique Facial Feature.

In our modern day, your Peeps are important to you because they'll be honest with you. Remember that their job is to keep you safe. They'll tell you what your Beautiful Unique Facial Feature is. All you need do is ask them. They'll let you know when it's not safe for you to look at social media because it'll further exacerbate your feelings of poor self-worth. They'll also tell you who you need to avoid following, watching, or having a relationship with and what you need to avoid doing. In this space, quietly, the people your Peeps feel you should follow will filter into your subconscious. The things your Peeps feel you should do will seep soothingly into your mind too. Before you know it, you're doing and letting into your life only the people and things enriching your life.

## Too much of a good thing is definitely a bad thing.

When you look at yourself in the mirror, it might be challenging to know what *your* unique facial feature is, but I promise you have one. If your face is untreated or you've had suitable treatments, you will often only have one unique facial feature. If you've had harmful injectable treatments, then sadly, you may have more than one. Your eyes, lips, jaw angle, chin, and smooth, wrinkle-free face might *all* be your unique facial features. Despite thinking that having more than one unique facial feature is a good thing, too much of a good thing is most definitely a bad thing.

Do you know why it's not a good thing? It creates confusion. Where do I look, what do I focus on? How would I describe that person to another? How do I compliment them?

"You have the most beautiful eyes," no longer seems appropriate when someone's lips are now disproportionate to their face and detract from their eyes.

## How do you find your Unique Facial Feature?

Think about someone you know, visualise their face, and then let your mind's eye wander to their Beautiful Unique Facial Feature. Naturally, your mind will go directly to it because it's also how you recognise and recall that person. The feature you might use when describing that person to another is their Beautiful Unique Facial Feature. It might be something you consider beautiful, like their eyes, or it might be something you would describe as quirky, cute, or unique. It's the facial feature that, if they no longer had it, they would no longer look like them.

Think of Jennifer Grey. One thing we loved so much about her was her nose. It made her unique and incredibly beautiful—like Barbra Streisand, who also has a prominent natural nose. If asked to describe Barbra Streisand to someone, but you couldn't remember her name, you'd likely say, "You know, great singer, unique nose, Lady Gaga played the same character in that movie..."

If you find it uncomfortable to look at yourself in the mirror, think about you in your early to mid-twenties and remember how people described and complimented you. Did they compliment you on your beautiful eyes, amazing eyelashes, stunning hair, incredible cheekbones, cute chin, lovely nose, or sweet lips?

When you're feeling *lost in your looks*, it's hard to remember anything positive that's ever been said about your appearance. You can quickly spiral downward into self-hate when you think about your appearance. So, this is a tough ask, I know it is, but give it a glancing thought while you cast your mind back to a younger you. The first thing that comes to mind about your face that others complimented you on, that is likely your Unique Facial Feature.

If you are only in your late teens or early 20s, you can use the above technique to find your Unique Facial Feature. Think about which of your facial features you receive the most compliments. What is it? That is your Unique Facial Feature.

I'd rather you didn't ask someone to tell you your unique facial feature. It's opening you up to judgement and can potentially destroy your self-confidence in a heartbeat. You must get through this part with only your Peeps (and me) guiding you.

## Don't ask for help, it can destroy you.

Two years ago, I had my self-confidence battered in precisely this way. After finding each other's unique facial feature, two colleagues were given the task of identifying mine. They took their time scrutinising my face, which was confronting enough. Finally, one gave up.

"I don't know," she said.

The other said, "It's tough. I think it might be your jaw, but I can't tell."

It devastated me. I'd always been complimented on my eyes, so I assumed they were my unique facial feature. But, in that instant, my eyes weren't worthy of praise. There was nothing unique about any of my normal-looking features. I thanked them for their assessment. I excused myself to the bathroom where I patted the tears from my insignificant eyes.

Years later, I'm still intrigued by this interaction, but I can justify it with my experience and education. So please, resist the temptation to ask someone what your Unique Facial Feature is for now. Deep down, *you know what it is anyway*. Ask your little Peeps inside you what your feature is, ask them, and be silent. Let them answer you. They will. You know the feature that made a potential partner go weak at the knees. You know your go-to feature that you make up when getting ready for a hot date or a night out.

I understand that during the above exercise you will probably think about all the things you hated most about your face when you were in your late teens and twenties. Still, we're not thinking about those here. Thank your mind for reminding you about them (therefore trying to protect you from further hurt caused by them) and move straight on to remembering the feature people most loved about your face. Write your Unique Facial Feature down, lock it in your brain for now.

## Step 2. Tapping and Emotional Freedom Technique

Emotional Freedom Technique is a meridian–based energy therapy, developed by Gary Craig (**https://www.emofree.com/eft-tutorial/eft-tapping-tutorial.html** 8/6/2020). In essence, we tap on the meridian points used for acupuncture.

It's a beneficial technique if you're having trouble appreciating your unique beauty or struggling with self-esteem and confidence issues.

I've been using Tapping as a great way to interrupt negative thought patterns and ground me. I use it regularly in conjunction with chatting with my Peeps. I ask my Peeps what is going on with them, what they are concerned about, and then I tap on that thing.

A brief outline of the method:

Holding your right-hand pointer and middle finger together, tap on each of the areas described below.

1. Karate chop (right-hand pointer and middle finger together and tap the underside edge of your left hand).
2. Between the eyebrows (hairy brow).
3. The temple (wise temple).
4. Beneath the eye (teardrop).
5. Beneath the nose (moustache).
6. On the chin (beard).
7. Beneath the collar bone.
8. Below the armpit.
9. Top of the head.

Here is a sample script to say to yourself while you tap with your right-hand pointer and middle finger together on all the nine points described above.

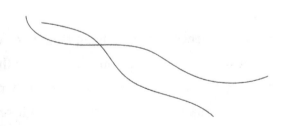

> *"Even though my... (insert facial feature you currently dislike, makes me feel like...) I deeply and completely love and accept myself."*
>
> Below are some examples of what you could say.
>
> *"Even though my...* **Lips are small,** *I deeply and completely love and accept myself..."*
>
> *"Even though my...* **Lips are uneven,** *I deeply and completely love and accept myself..."*
>
> *"Even though my...* **Nose is too big,** *I deeply and completely love and accept myself..."*
>
> Nose is a weird shape.
>
> Eyes are deep-set.
>
> Eyes are small.
>
> Forehead is big.

You get the idea! It will get you over the hump of focusing on the parts of your face that distract you from your Unique Facial Feature.

Do the cycle of Tapping a few times or until you experience a feeling of release.

You might experience sadness, anger, happiness, or a moment of clarity about what is bothering you when you do this exercise.

For example, when I did this activity in the writing of this book, up came a situation that happened in high school, which I thought I'd forgotten. I was about fourteen years old, and a group of older boys walked past me. One of them said, "Great body, shame about the face." Well, this event came back like a thunderclap when I started Tapping about my Unique Facial Feature. I don't know why, but it did. I visualised myself as that impressionable young woman and the effect that one comment made on my self-esteem for the rest of my life. And then I tapped about that.

*"Even though that boy hurt me with his comment, I deeply and completely love and accept myself."*

*"Even though he said I had an ugly face, I deeply and completely love and accept myself."*

*"Even though that boy's comment has made me feel ugly for the last thirty years, I deeply and completely love and accept myself."*

I then forgave the boy for saying it, and I forgave myself for believing it for thirty years.

Think about the Unique Facial Feature you've identified and written in a journal or notepad. Beneath it, write down all the beautiful things anyone has ever said about your face.

"Your eyes are such an interesting colour."

"Your skin is so lovely and clear."

"Your eyes are such a pretty shape."

Don't stop to think or edit yourself; just write whatever comes into your mind.

I saw a social media post that sums up exactly what I want you to do now.

> *"The best thing for a woman's self-esteem is drunk women complimenting her in the bathroom on a night out."* How true is this?! When we're tipsy, we vocalise the lovely things we see in other women. Be one of those complimenting women now. Write out all the things that are unique and lovely about your face.

## Step 3. Mantra - I love myself.

At my most desperate and ill point in 2019, it didn't matter how many times the people I cared about told me they loved me. The more love they showered on me, the more I felt I was unworthy of their love. I'd spiral into further guilt and self-loathing. Without making my patients, husband, daughters, family, and friends happy, I wasn't worthy. Without making everything perfect for them, I wasn't worthy. I realised there was no way I could feel loved if I didn't love and accept myself first.

After my blow up/meltdown/break down/burnout/near-death experience of 2019, I started telling myself, "I love you." I would place my hand on a part of my body (often across my heart,) close my eyes, and say, "I love you." It worked well in halting the feelings I had of not living up to my expectations of myself. It still does. But I found I could improve it.

When the first draft of this book was with the editor, I stumbled across Kamal Ravikant's book, 'Love Yourself Like Your Life Depends on it.' (https://kamal.blog) 8/6/2020. In it, I learned something valuable that could apply to my learnings and help my readers, too.

Kamal Ravikant also hit rock bottom and, from it, created his vow; "I love myself." It was exciting to read that someone else felt brave enough to tell the world that they, too, learned to say to themselves that they loved themselves. I found sometimes my version of "I love you" backfired. Depending on where I was at when I said it, my mind quickly wandered to the people in my life that I say "I love you" to the most: my daughters and my husband. I'd say, "I love you," intending to tell myself that I loved myself. Still, most of the time, my mind would go down the familiar neural pathway of guilt, so I would end up feeling guilty about being a bad mum and a bad wife. Thanks to Kamal Ravikant, I started to experiment with, "I love myself" and "I love you."

## Look for the heroes. Look for the beauty.

Once I saw the beauty in me and, by this I don't just mean physical beauty but also emotional beauty; I found I could see more beauty in others, too. Tell it to your children if you see something beautiful, say it to yourself, say it to others. Start complimenting people, places, and things. Feel the joy that giving compliments also gives you. Always look for beauty. With this behaviour you encourage others to do the same. If you can't find the beauty, then change the scenery.

I developed anxiety from losing sight of beauty. Looking for the proof that I was failing, disappointing and upsetting those around me, meant I couldn't see the beauty any longer. I see this pattern in my patients all the time. It's easy to stop seeing the beauty in the world because we first stop seeing the beauty in ourselves. By looking for external verification only, we expect the world to make us feel joy when it is our responsibility to find joy within ourselves. 'I love myself.'

Every day, multiple times a day, and whenever you feel you need to get out of a mindset rut, do the Inner Power Practice. 1. Peeps, 2. Tapping, and 3. Mantra. The effect on you is wondrous.

## INNER POWER PRACTICE

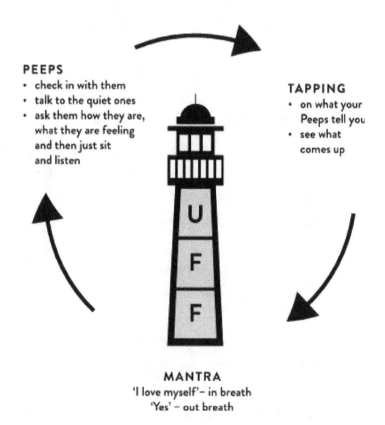

**PEEPS**
- check in with them
- talk to the quiet ones
- ask them how they are, what they are feeling and then just sit and listen

**TAPPING**
- on what your Peeps tell you
- see what comes up

U
F
F

**MANTRA**
'I love myself'– in breath
'Yes' – out breath

**Anchors:**

There are three anchors to keep you safe in the connection you have to your lighthouse - Unique Facial Feature (UFF) and your Beautiful Unique Face (BUF)

**1. Peeps**. Check in with them. Breathe with them on the wave of your breath. Ask them if they're ok? Listen to the quiet ones. What are they saying? Are they happy and relaxed? Are they distracted? What are they feeling? Remember, these can be big or small things. Everything they tell you is crucial.

**2. Tapping** about the things your Peeps are telling you. If they're worried about something you have planned for your day, tap it out. If they're unsure about the dress you're planning on wearing, tap it out. If they're worried about someone, tap about them. See what comes up and tap about it until you get to the bottom of it, and it feels clearer.

**3. Mantra**. "I love myself" Now take ten deep breaths in and out. On your in breath say, "I love myself," and on your out breath say, "Yes."

Remember, you can do these without anyone knowing. You don't need to be in a private place. You can tap discreetly. It's fun to watch your mindset change as a direct result of doing these three anchors.

CASE STUDY: LINDY

## "I feel less attractive than I used to. I feel less feminine, too."

Lindy had been a patient of mine for eighteen months. During our initial consultation, Lindy told me her main concern was her frown and forehead lines, and the excess fat under her chin. We perform a fat-dissolving treatment in my clinic, and Lindy was interested, saying she'd recently been told she looked like her father.

*"I feel less attractive than I used to. I feel less feminine, too."*

After examining Lindy's face and hearing her concerns, I discussed what I saw happening to her face. As a forty-four-year-old woman, Lindy's face had undergone some significant changes as she'd aged.

We lose our facial fat pads and our face shows signs of ageing from the age of twenty-seven when our oestrogen starts to decline. Our oestrogen continues to decline, and evidence of facial ageing becomes more apparent by the age of 40, 50, 60, and beyond.

Lindy felt that, since her 40th birthday, she'd looked much older, and her face strongly resembled her father's. It was highly likely. We do look more like our parents, generally one parent more than the other, after our 40th birthday. All thanks to our face mimicking the way our parent's face has aged. If it is a prominent chin that our parent has, that's what we tend to develop. It's the way our genetics has already dictated how members of our family age.

Lindy had a lovely, kind, open, and calming face. Her frown and forehead (aka worry) lines were strong and etched into her skin. Her cheek fat pads had descended slightly, creating slight jowls, and her chin had lifted slightly. It meant her face looked square and, indeed, somewhat masculine. I discussed Lindy's face shape and part of the reason she saw under chin fat (which we all have, but it increases as we age) was that her chin was becoming shorter.

## We often feel good about ourselves until we catch a glimpse of ourselves.

Lindy had a great sense of humour. She was bright and sassy. And she felt her face was no longer representing how she felt inside. I understood the mismatch between how she felt inside and what she saw in the mirror. We often feel good about ourselves until we catch a glimpse of ourselves or someone comments on the way we are looking. "You look tired." "What's wrong? You look upset." It can be confusing and confidence destroying when we receive comments meant to present concern, but only make us feel bad about ourselves. These offhand comments confirm a belief that we have about our face; we're not beautiful.

I empathised with Lindy and agreed it is hard when we feel good in ourselves, but we think our face conveys a different message. I explained we would use Botox to treat her frown and worry lines.

*"The lines have become etched into your skin just like when you fold a piece of paper over and over. It creates a crease where the fold has been. It's why your frown and worry lines are there when you are not frowning or feeling worried."*

Sometimes the lines are so deeply etched into a patient's skin that I cannot fully lift them and smooth the skin. The wrinkle lines can become like scars in the skin, and the skin changes at a cellular level.

*"Muscle relaxant treatment into your frown and forehead area*

*forces you to stop folding that piece of paper over and over. While I'm not sure if we'll completely lift the lines, we will soften them and make them less obvious," I explained.*

*Lindy needed to understand the limitations of the treatment, so she had realistic expectations of her result. Lindy still wanted to know about the fat-dissolving treatment for under her chin. "Can I dissolve this fat here?"*

Like many of us, sometimes we need someone else to examine us and tell us what's happening with our face. All Lindy could see was the fat under her chin area. She didn't realise the reason it was suddenly more apparent to her was that not only had it likely increased in size, but her chin was lifted thanks to the increased strength of the chin muscle. It led to the overall square look that Lindy was noticing in her lower face.

*"We can certainly dissolve what fat is there, but we'd ideally do some dermal filler in your chin first. It'll feminise your chin and create softer curves. It'll help to reduce the heaviness in your lower face."*

*"I don't want dermal fillers," Lindy replied.*

Like many women, Lindy was worried about having dermal fillers. She felt it was a step too far.

*"I don't want fillers. I don't want to look like those women who are all puffy and look weird. That's from fillers, isn't it?"*

*"It's from dermal fillers done badly. You wouldn't look like that. I don't allow that to happen in my practice, Lindy. I am an advocate of normality."*

Lindy was worried she would become a PUF. In light of what is happening in today's society, it was a reasonable fear to have.

During the next eighteen months, although always her witty, sassy, and kind self, Lindy felt something was missing.

*"I just don't feel feminine any longer."*

*She had her hair cut very short and stopped wearing dresses and makeup.*

*"I feel like I look like a bloke," Lindy said.*

A sensitive topic, this came up every time I saw Lindy. Each time we discussed the chin treatment I'd recommended initially, and each time Lindy refused.

*"I don't want fillers. I don't want to look like those women who are all puffy and look weird. That's from fillers, isn't it?"*

It took months of regular treatment for Lindy's frown, forehead, and chin with Botox for her to trust me enough to let me perform a chin augmentation for her. As I performed the treatment, something remarkable happened I didn't expect. As I made Lindy's square lower face fade into the background, her eyes came out of nowhere making me feel like I'd been punched firmly on the nose.

## I'd been fooled.

How had I missed the deep, dark, almost black colour of her eyes all this time? So fixated on her chin, whenever I'd seen her, that's all I'd seen. I'd never noticed her Unique Facial Feature, her almost-onyx coloured eyes. Her eyes had always been the lead actor of her face, but her square chin pulling focus, had me fooled.

It took me twenty minutes to complete the treatment and, when I finished, I handed Lindy the mirror. She shook her head, shocked. Tears filled her huge, exquisite eyes.

I saw Lindy at her next scheduled appointment three months later. She told me a story so poignant it made it into this book. Her lesson warmed me to the core. It reminded me why our unique facial feature is the key to unlocking our true happiness and fully growing into our Beautiful Unique Face.

Once Lindy left my clinic after having her chin augmentation, she said she felt more feminine than she had in a long time. On that drive home, while still euphoric from seeing herself in the mirror in my clinic, Lindy called her and her husband's favourite restaurant and made a booking for that evening.

*"I arranged a babysitter, got dressed in my husband's favourite dress, put some makeup on, and my husband and I went out for a date night. For the first time in a long time, I felt like a woman again. I've felt feminine ever since. Thank you."*

*"Oh, Lindy. I'm so happy." I said.*

*"Why did I wait so long?" she asked.*

*"You needed to be ready," I replied.*

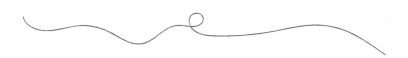

# Part Two

# ONE TO TWO STEPS AHEAD.

## CASE STUDY: DIANNE

Dianne first entered my clinic looking like a scared and lost puppy dog. She was ashamed and embarrassed just to be sitting in my waiting room. Her her tail firmly between her legs.

I recognised the signs. Women who have minimal self-worth always look like this. I want to bundle them up straight away in a warm embrace and tell them it's ok; they are safe, and I will look after them. Dianne looked at me suspiciously when I said her name, another typical trait of a woman who has nothing left in her tank. It's almost as though the last shred of dignity has gone out the window because they're seeking help from a Botox clinic, the last place they ever imagined themselves being.

*Dianne couldn't look me in the eye.*

*After the pleasantries, Dianne could see that I was a nice and, most importantly, a normal-looking woman. I asked her how I could help.*

*"I'm looking old and horrible."*

*"How old are you?"*

*"I'm sixty-nine, but I look older than sixty-nine. I think I look eighty."*

I examined Dianne's face while she talked. She still hadn't held my gaze and looked to the ground as she was talking.

**"I'm being vain, aren't I?"**

*"I've become obsessed with looking at other women my age and comparing myself to them. When I see a woman my age, I know I look worse than them, and it can put me on a downer for days, even weeks. Then no one truly knows what is wrong with me and why I'm upset. It can make me cranky, especially at my husband."*

"Oh, Dianne, I understand. I truly do."

"When people ask me what's wrong, I'm too embarrassed to say what is bothering me. I'm scared if I tell someone, they'll say I'm stupid or vain."

"I understand."

"The only reason I'm here is, I think it's making me depressed. I wouldn't be here otherwise. I think those ladies who have all this stuff done to their faces look stupid."

"You're very brave to have even made the appointment to see me, Dianne."

"You're the only person who knows how I feel about my face. I hate my skin. I've never really taken great interest in my appearance because I always felt ugly. I've never worn makeup. I feel silly in makeup, like a clown trying to hide my face. And I just feel like it draws more attention to my face. That's the last thing I want, attention drawn to my face. I've always been slim and active, always played sports, and like to be outdoors, which is why my skin is so bad. I've so much sun damage. I've had skin cancers cut out from my face."

We moved onto what Dianne hoped to achieve from our session.

"I want to do something for me, not for anyone else. I don't want anyone to notice I've had anything done. You won't make me look like those ladies whose faces look horrible, will you?"

"I can promise you, Dianne; I won't make you look overdone. No one will notice you've had anything done, they'll just see that you look well and refreshed."

"I don't even know what I can have done. If there is anything that can make me look any better, anyway. I just thought I would come and ask…"

"Yes, I have a plan. I have been watching while you talk and already have an excellent idea about what we can do to help you."

"I'm stupid, aren't I?" Dianne began to cry. "My husband would be furious if he knew I was here. He'd tell me not to be silly, and that I was being vain. But it's for me, not anyone else."

"You are most definitely not being stupid or vain, Dianne. You are brave and strong and doing something to help yourself, which will consequently improve your relationship with yourself and others. You're very courageous," I said.

I continued. "Let's talk about your Beautiful Unique Facial Feature. Your cheekbones are naturally beautiful. You are incredibly lucky to have such amazing cheekbones."

I introduced Dianne to her Unique Facial Feature for the first time, surprised to find that Dianne had always felt that her sharp cheekbones made her look gaunt and sickly.

"People feel it's ok to comment that I look too thin all the time. Certain people say every time I see them, that I've lost more weight. But I haven't. I haven't lost weight. Every time they say that, it makes me feel like they're saying I look ugly."

*"To have natural cheekbones like yours, Dianne, is exceptional. It means we have a wonderful foundation with which to work. I create cheekbones like yours in people who don't have them. You have them naturally. There's no beating that."*

We finished our discussion and made a plan to enhance Dianne's Unique Facial Feature so that her face looked natural and normal and that the audience focused on her 'lead actor,' her nature-gifted cheekbones. Then we carried out the first part of the treatment. I handed Dianne the mirror at the end.

*"Wow, I never knew this was possible. I look so much better already. Thank you."*

*"Keep in mind that your muscle relaxants haven't kicked in yet. They take the full two weeks to take effect. Also, the dermal fillers that you can see now will take two weeks to settle fully. So that's why I'll see you in two weeks for a review."*

## One to two steps ahead.

I believe we look for people who we think are 1-2 steps ahead of us, to inspire and lead us. These people often appear to have their life more together than we do. They've achieved success both professionally and personally in areas that hold value for us. We can imagine ourselves living their lives without too much difficulty. Looking to these people, we can fantasise about standing in their shoes in the not too distant future. Without realising it, we look to these people to help guide our decisions in a great many things. They are not as untouchable as royalty or mythical beings. The people who are 1-2 steps ahead have lives that we can easily imagine as our own.

## Please look after us, for we need to be led.

We need to be led. We like to feel like someone else has been there before us and survived. And we need to feel like someone else knows what's going on, will take care of us, and make the critical decisions in the world. In times gone by, these were the gods, but now they are celebrities and politicians. All of whom are simply humans trying to forge their way in life. Not unlike ourselves.

I repeat, we need to be led. It is why influencers can rack up thousands upon thousands of followers. It's not because they are saying anything profound or even motivating us to be better humans. It's because we need someone to look up to, and they are happy to share everything with us. In this digital age, when face-to-face interaction is declining, it's how we feel like we're not alone.

## Who's leading you?

Before social media was a massive part of our lives, we looked to films, magazines, and TV for aspirational people. In a way, it was safer. The celebrities in movies were people we couldn't really imagine being like. They were of a completely different league. Untouchable. Once reality TV shows came into our houses (Kardashians), we saw behind the scenes of relatively normal people who slept like us, ate like us, loved like us and felt the same fears and joys as us. This changed the perception of what we could achieve. Suddenly, we no longer looked to the A-list celebrities we always knew were out-of-reach, but now looked to the reality TV stars for inspiration. Once we imagined ourselves being like them, it was easy to imagine us experiencing the things they did.

Injectable treatments now shown in our very own lounge room via the TV seemed to hurt only a teeny bit. People looked so good and were so happy afterward. We wanted that, too. And, before too long, we could have it.

Botox and dermal filler treatments were suddenly more accessible. No longer a treatment reserved for the untouchable rich and famous. Still, it was getting closer to being within our reach too. Then came social media, especially Instagram, where everyone is an 'influencer' with not only an opinion but something to sell.

We all know a 'normal' person who has become an influencer overnight, with a considerable following and ability to impact the lives of the people who 'follow' them. Heck, I'm trying to influence your thought patterns here. Influencers are now the people who are easily 1-2 steps ahead of us. Most definitely within our reach and absolutely someone we can aspire to look like and behave similarly to. I don't know about you, but I often wonder how on earth people who have nothing but utter rot to say are 'influencers' and have so much clout in my world. I despise the term and the notion behind it. I am so relieved I no longer work as a full-time actor or TV presenter. I would be competing not only against my fellow creatives but also with every person who decided that they wanted to be an overnight sensation.

## Take charge of who you put one to two steps ahead of you.

It's not the fault of your smartphone if you can't be without it. It's also not the fault of social media that you feel inadequate unless you have the lips an influencer; it's advertising.

If you're reading this book, you're an adult and have the choice to take charge of your actions. Choose to act a certain way. The way you'd act if you wholeheartedly loved yourself. Don't react the instant you see something. Let it sit in your mind and body. Let it sit in your heart. Take your time to respond. Ask your Peeps what they think about it. Ask your Peeps to think about the feeling that you're experiencing. Be picky; be choosey. It is, after all, your life.

Ask your Peeps, does this person who is selling me this idea align with my values? Does the way they behave reflect my values? Then listen for the answer.

The people we put 1–2 steps ahead of us, the people we aspire to be like in our life, we place in hugely influential positions. Make sure these people are worthy of their position. Choose wisely because, subconsciously, you will become them whether you like it or not. Instead of trying to mirror someone else, turn the mirror around and look to yourself for the guidance you need. Remember, your Peeps are your very own cheer squad. They know you better than you know yourself. They want you to win. They adore you.

## Be your own hero.

Here's a novel thought, put *yourself* 1–2 steps ahead. Not anyone else. Given that these days we often look to questionable sources for our inspiration, I think this is by far the safest thing to do. Use them only as examples of where you can go, but not to the detriment of your self-esteem. Stop comparing yourself to them and thinking you will not be enough until you're like them. It will only ever make you feel perpetually inadequate. Be the one you want to be more like. Be your own hero.

The problem we all have today is trying to mimic other people who we believe are better than us. *We* are the best person for us. We are enough, and when you believe this, you will smash through any limitations you have on your ability to be better. Being the best version of yourself is trendy right now with terms like 'live your best life', 'live your truth'. But we can be left wondering, what on earth this actually is and how do we even get there?

## Tap it out.

Tap about any insecurities that come up when you consider making yourself your very own hero. They may sound like this; 'I can't be my own hero because..."

*"I'm too young, too old, too short, too tall, I have a stupid voice, I'm in loads of debt, I don't have a job, I don't have a partner, I have a messy wardrobe, I have a pimple, I need to get petrol, I cried this morning, I have a bloated tummy, I forgot to call my mum, I'm too tired, I have nothing I want to do, I have too many things to do, I don't know anything."*

As you can see, the list is endless. In an effort for self-preservation, we'll conjure up any excuse to convince ourselves that we're not enough. We need to look to someone else to make us worthy.

Let's make the Tapping script, "Even though I can't be my own hero because I don't know anything, I deeply and completely love and accept myself."

See where this takes you now. My Tapping journey went like this. "Even though I'm not a hero...

> *"Even though I don't know anything worthy..."*
> *"Even though I can't possibly lead myself..."*
> *"Even though I'm lost..."*
> *"Even though I have no one to help me..."*
> *"Even though everyone will think I'm up myself..."*
> *and then finish your Tapping script with, "I deeply and completely love and accept myself."*

I got sick because I was trying to make it perfect for everyone else by doing something for them. So obsessed with perfection myself, I even made it my business value statement. Women approached me wanting to look more beautiful but were petrified of looking fake and overdone. I also had many women approaching me already over-treated and miserable with the way they looked. Yet, they were now firmly stuck on the hamster wheel, and they felt they couldn't get off. These women believed that the only option was to be unhappy with how they looked before treatment or unhappy with their over-treated faces after treatment. Both groups of women desperately wanted to find the secret to their unique beauty. Both groups of women believed that perfection was something they could achieve.

DIANNE CONTINUED.
A few weeks later, Dianne returned. She was like a different woman sitting in my waiting room this time around. Relaxed and calm, Dianne unleashed her beautiful smile on me as I ushered her into my treatment room.

*Gushing, she said, "I'm so happy. No one noticed! Only my*

*grandson said one day, 'Nanna, you look beautiful.' He broke my heart. I cried and hugged him tightly. No one has ever told me I look beautiful."*

It was incredible how we were able to change Dianne's extremely negative mindset about herself by introducing her to her Unique Facial Feature.

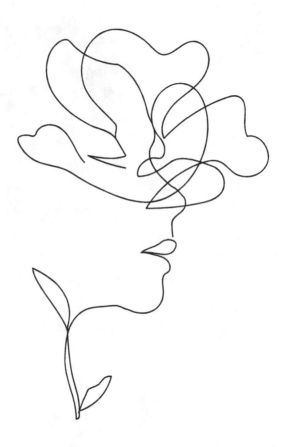

# Chapter Four

## Part One

## INNER POWER PRACTICE.

CASE STUDY: SANDY

**"I can't do it anymore. I can't cope. Somehow, I do it all, and I'm the envy of everyone. I'm everything to everybody but nothing to myself. I'm a fraud."**

Sandy is the artistic director of a successful marketing firm where she'd worked for ten years. Her hard work and expert creative flair brought the company back from the brink of bankruptcy. It now stood as an award-winning multinational company, boasting some excellent businesses amongst its clients. Sandy was an admired and passionate director to her team and a well-respected member of the business. That was until she and her team won the contract of the company's dreams. She excused herself from the celebrations. In the bathroom, Sandy looked at her reflection in the mirror.

## The following is Sandy's recollection of the events that unfolded on that day.

*"I'm so lonely. I'm so sad. I'm confused. Here I am, the praise of my colleagues, but I don't feel good enough. I'm not worthy of their praise."*

*I cry.*

*"I can't do it anymore. I can't cope. Somehow, I do it all, and I'm the envy of everyone. I'm everything to everybody but nothing to myself. I'm a fraud. My kids have grown up; I've never been around to mother them. My husband, a man I don't even see anymore. We don't talk. He sits on his laptop working and I sit on mine. I haven't looked at him in months, and I'm sure he hasn't looked at me. I've always worked and been busy. I'm always so bloody busy."*

*I feel a choking sensation in my throat and think I might vomit. I lift the toilet seat and see the evidence of the woman who used the toilet before me.*

*"Who was she? Did she feel like me? Does anyone else feel like this? I feel so full and yet so empty. I sit on the toilet and turn on my phone. I contemplate calling my husband to tell him about the contract win, but don't. Is he even in the country at the moment?"*

*I open Instagram instead. I scroll through images of friends and women I've never met. How in control, relaxed and, quite frankly, perfect they all look. Whether having fun with their family, or focused and respected at work, or out celebrating with friends, they look happy and gorgeous. I leave the cubical. In the mirror, my makeup-smudged face peers back at me.*

*"Look at you. You're a joke, a fraud, try to smile, try to hide by burying yourself deeper in your work. You're ugly. You're old. Mere*

*moments away from losing your husband, your kids, and your self-respect. Your children used to look up to you; they used to love you so much their bodies ached for yours."*

*Instead of nurturing my children, being the perfect mother and housewife, I've been busy forging my way in my indulgent career. Why couldn't I be satisfied with being a wife and mother?*

*"Are you too good for that? Who would you have disappointed if you were the mother you now wish you'd been? Who made you this way? This drive to sacrifice everyone else happiness, so that you could be the head of the company. Earn the big bucks. Earn the big respect."*

*"Well, guess what? The tell-tale signs are showing. The lines around your lips are poor at hiding the secrets you keep buried deep inside. Darkened hollows beneath your eyes that your concealer struggles to cover. You're starting to show the gaping cracks in your bleeding soul and the tears of uncertainty you shed in the shower. The crevices etched in between your eyebrows tell the fear that wafts into the nostrils of others as you walk by. Your head full of frustration, held high. Your forehead tells of the worry we know wakes you with a start at 2am every morning. The 2am mirror that hovers perilously close to your face, reflecting your disintegrating and sad life. Sometimes a broken mirror, its shards of glass, showing you all the failings that you are today, anticipating all the failings you will make in the future and disappointment you have inflicted on others throughout your life.*

*Gut-wrenching worry that you're about to be found out as the fraud you are. Worry that you're about to lose control once and for all. Your seemingly perfect life will come crashing down. Someone younger will surpass you, brighter, wittier, fitter, and way more attractive than you are. The skin on your body is loose now. Marked with lines and unsightly brown spots. You need a new wardrobe, full of clothes for a worn out, burnt out, tired and washed-up old woman.*

I look down at my aching feet. Every big client dinner and meeting I attend; I wear these 'special' high heels.

*"You think you look glamorous. Seriously, you do. You honestly think you look good in those shoes. A man at last year's conference in Paris told you these shoes made your legs look amazing. Flattered, you bought two more pairs online the next day."*

He was probably joking. I was drunk after all. Dancing all sexy with him. I'm too old to dance. I'm so embarrassed. I remember it now. Oh no, why didn't I see then that he was mocking me? In that moment, I felt human and alive, and like someone saw me, the once gorgeous, sexy and desirable woman that I once was. Then life took hold and shook it all out of me.

*"Now I'm reminding you of him, of your interaction with him that night, you're embarrassed. And yes, you should be. The horror. Don't be confused. Are you angry? Who are you angry with?"*

Sandy looked down at her swollen feet and kicked off her shoes. Big important tender meeting this morning. Needed to win the contract. Pulled out the 'special' shoes the French cutie said I looked sexy wearing. Bile comes up into my mouth.

I have no idea why the incident in Paris has come hurtling at me like a runaway train. I keep scrolling through Instagram. I'm feeling worse with every post I see.

*"Wipe your eyes, wipe your nose, wipe the sadness from your face. Wipe away the lipstick bleeding into the lines around your mouth. Wipe the eye shadow away from the old lady skin creases of your eyelids. Wipe the misery from your face, get back to your office, and make some important decisions. Oh, and by the way, call this number. Get some Botox into those lines. Sort those thin scowling*

*lips out. Get some volume into your cheeks and turn that permanent mouth scowl upside down. SORT YOUR FACE OUT."*

## Inner power practice.

When we discuss anchors in psychological terms, we refer to a well-rehearsed pattern of belief that then informs our decision making. There are healthy and unhealthy anchors. For example, "I am not as smart as my brother, therefore, there is no way that I can work out that complex math problem." "I have curly hair, therefore, there is no way that I can ever have long flowing locks." "I had bad skin as a teenager, therefore, there is no way that I can ever believe someone when they compliment my complexion."

Your anchors are formed early in your life and often mirror those of your family. Families carry anchors from past generations and are usually about money, behaviour, relationships, status, and self-worth. Anchors can be self-limiting and damaging, or they can be liberating and self-loving.

Unbeknownst to us, one of our very first anchors after our birth is our Unique Facial Feature. We get complimented on our eyes, or our cheeks, or our lips, or our smile. Whatever stands out when we are toddlers, and is what we get complimented on, is our Unique Facial Feature.

As children, we know how to use our Unique Facial Feature because we have learned that's what draws people to us. It gives us what we need as much as food, water, and shelter - love. It's what our personality is intrinsically shaped by. Our cheeky smile ignites our cheeky and fun personality. Our deep, dark eyes are what give our mysterious character the foundation on which to grow.

Our features are described with emotion-evoking words, better placed describing a physical thing. It shows how our Unique Facial

Feature informs our personality. Otherwise, surely, we would describe a smile as large rather than bright, a jaw as poking out rather than handsome and strong. It's another reason people with over-treated faces lose their ability to connect with others.

Along the journey of life, we lose focus on our Unique Facial Feature. By the time we are teenagers and young adults and firmly focused on everything but our Unique Facial Feature. Telling ourselves, *'I'm not enough,'* and that pathway in our brain gets well-worn and predictable.

Predictability, for most, means comfort. If we know, or have a fairly accurate expectation of, how something will play out it won't shock us when it happens the way we've anticipated. But choose your pathway well. Make your familiar and predictable pathway one that opens up your world to possibility and lets you flourish.

We continue to look outside of ourselves for insight into what makes us beautiful when no other human being on earth has the exact Unique Facial Feature. Just like fingerprints, no two are the same.

INNER POWER PRACTICE

**PEEPS**
• check in with them
• talk to the quiet ones
• ask them how they are, what they are feeling and then just sit and listen

**TAPPING**
• on what your Peeps tell you
• see what comes up

U
F
F

**MANTRA**
'I love myself'– in breath
'Yes' – out breath

> If our Unique Facial Feature is the key to our beauty, it seems odd then, that we'd try to mirror anyone else. For we are not them and they are not us.

It's why I've made your Unique Facial Feature the lighthouse of all you need to carry on forwards and upwards in your wondrous and loving life ahead.

Women love the idea of their Unique Facial Feature being their lighthouse. Chosen because of its nautical theme, stoic classic beauty and role to protect all who look to it in times of trouble, your lighthouse serves to secure our anchors; Peeps, Tapping and Mantra.

Your Unique Facial Feature is the always dependable and robust rod that stands within you, supporting you and keeping you on course throughout your life. Regardless of what external forces say is beautiful about you, your Unique Facial Feature, your lighthouse, is *your* key to *your* beauty.

## You choose your pathway.

With access to everyone else's lives through the media and social media, it's easy to compare ourselves to others. We gauge our place in the world based on those around us. Through the eyes of comparison, we see something that makes us feel unworthy. We quickly judge ourselves unfairly.

The way our neural pathways work is this. The more we think a specific thought, the more well-worn and clearer that walking path becomes. It's easier for us to walk down that neural path without stumbling. Thinking a negative thought about ourselves or others is easier to do than thinking a positive thought. It's what needs to change. You choose your pathway.

Stand in front of two doorways. Open the door to the path on your right first. See a well-lit walking path ahead. Now fill it with all of your favourite sights and smells. The plants you love, your favourite flowers. Make it your favourite season and, at the end of the path, place the most comfortable seat. This walking path is the most beautiful path you have ever seen in your life. It gives you the happiest feeling as you gaze down at it.

Now, open the door to the path on your left. In it, there is fire, evil, and fear. All the things that make you horrified, angry and helpless cover this walking path. The plants are stingers, and the animals are biters. The season is your most loathed time of year. At the end of this path sits the greatest fear in your life waiting— something that you'd protect your family and friends from ever experiencing.

If someone asked you to choose between the paths, 100% of the time you'd select the door opening to the beautiful path. It's the path you travel down every time you complete the Mantra and feel self-love.

The ugly path sees you full of self-loathing and belief that you're not good enough. It's the path of hell. You'd never open the door if given a choice between the two. Yet so often, we find ourselves in an eternal cycle of self-loathing that sees us stuck on that pathway of hell.

Whenever you feel the external world pulling and pushing you down the evil path, dig your heels in and refuse to go. Instead, follow the beautiful pathway you've created with your Peeps, Tapping, and Mantra.

## It's your responsibility to know and respect your Unique Facial Feature.

It's not a level playing field out there anymore. We're compared by others and by ourselves to women who have and haven't had treatment. Sometimes the women who've had treatment look good because it's done well, and their Unique Facial Feature is carefully respected. Other times, because it's been done poorly, their Unique Facial Feature is overlooked, and they look over-treated.

One of the biggest misconceptions around having treatments done is that you're dammed if you do and you're dammed if you don't. It's no wonder that we put all our trust into the practitioner performing the treatment to keep us, not only medically safe, but also to look the best we can.

## It's why knowing your Unique Facial Feature is essential.

Better still is going to a practitioner who carefully considers your Unique Facial Feature and, based on it, establishes your treatment plan. It will ensure you will always look beautiful.

SANDY CONTINUED.

Sandy shared with me that she regularly travelled down the path of self-loathing. However, once she considered the two doors leading to either the pathway of love or the path of hate, she vowed to never knowingly travel down the path of hate again.

*Sandy was nervous about having treatment done.*

*"I've seen women who have had too much done, and I don't ever want to look like that," she said.*

*I understood completely. I ensure my patients are never over-treated.*

Sandy requested treatment for her frown lines, crow's feet wrinkles, and forehead lines. She also wanted dermal fillers to help lift the wrinkles around her mouth.

I identified that her Unique Facial Feature was her naturally high cheekbones, including the bone structure from her cheekbones up to her eyebrows. Sandy was fifty years old and had lost a small amount of volume in her face, which made her cheekbones look sharp with new hollows forming beneath them. It often happens to women with beautiful cheekbones and can lead to their faces looking hard and angular.

**Ageing isn't always kind to our faces. Still, without an appreciation of our lighthouse and three anchors, our minds can make the effects of ageing seem much worse.**

*"Yes, my cheekbones used to get compliments all the time. Now people treat me like I'm cranky, which in turn makes me cranky. I feel like being alone most of the time. I don't know what to do about it."*

*"We'll focus on your beautiful cheekbones. They've always been and will always be your Unique Facial Feature. We can tailor your treatments and mindset around keeping them as your focus, your lighthouse."*

*We softened the sharpness of Sandy's cheekbones and restored the curves she naturally had in her mid-face. It instantly took the focus off the hollowing beneath her cheekbones and restored her softer, more feminine appearance.*

*Sandy looked in the mirror.*

*"I look more like me now, it's strange. I didn't realise I'd stopped looking like me. Although, it explains it. I haven't felt like me for so long. I now feel settled," she said.*

*We put Botox in Sandy's frown and forehead lines to soften the negative lines that made her look 'cranky.' And we softened the wrinkles around her eyes. The small amount of light dermal filler we used to lift her lip lines was barely noticeable, just as we wanted.*

**"I look better, I know I do, but I don't feel any better."**

*I saw Sandy two weeks later, after her treatments kicked in and settled down.*

*"I look better, I know I do, but I don't feel any better."*

*"How do you feel?"*

*"I feel like other women are still happier than me. I expected once I knew what my Unique Facial Feature was, that I'd feel happy like them. And every time I looked in the mirror, I'd feel good."*

The women Sandy referred to were the women she saw on social media, not women she saw face to face in real life.

It's not a level playing field, and you can't possibly base your self-worth on images you see on social media. There are many things to consider here that play a massive role in making you compare yourself to others. Social media is not an accurate representation of someone's life at all times. It's merely a staged snapshot and as with any final performance, they've taken many rehearsals of that photo before it sees the light of day and you look at it on your phone.

Filters and face-changing apps are used endlessly in mainstream and social media. I've even seen photos posted stating they haven't used a filter when it's clear to anyone they have used one. Perhaps the right thing to accompany a photo like this is, "Not the normal level of filter has been applied to this photo."

No amount of stuff we inject into our faces, even when done well, or exercise we put our body through, or lovely clothes we wear, will address our internal happiness. Without doing the inner work and, if needed, seeing a professional to work through our feelings, can we expect to feel happy? Social media has a nasty habit of making you believe it can.

## Do the work.

It has taken a long time for my mindset to change, and it's only come about thanks to my doing the internal work. This is the work that serves as a constant reminder not to get sucked into social media and believe what my eyes tell my brain is real.

I focus on four trustworthy and reliable things, especially when my mind threatens to open the door to the pathway of evil. My lighthouse, my Peeps, my Tapping and my Mantra. Solid concepts that keep me positive, happy, and beautiful, inside and out.

In my clinic, the time we have allocated in an appointment can make it difficult to address the three anchors with the women I treat, so I educate them on their Unique Facial Feature. Their lighthouse is their foremost priority. Sometimes I will introduce them to their Peeps or Tapping or their Mantra. Depending on the woman and what I feel will work best for them.

I hope that with this book, everyone can learn to use their lighthouse and three anchors.

*"I find when I compare myself too much to others, Sandy, I need to remind myself of how loved I am by me. One of the ways I*

*do this is with my, 'I love myself. Yes.' Mantra."*

*I described to Sandy how I do this, and together we practiced it. Sandy had been judging herself harshly for such a long time. It was evident she needed reminding of how loved she was.*

*You wouldn't knowingly throw yourself down the path of fire and evil, but throw yourself down the path of self-love with as much enthusiasm and watch the positive changes happen.*

*"You deserve to look and feel beautiful, Sandy."*

Sandy left my clinic on that day, excited about her new sense of control over how she felt when she was overwhelmed by self-loathing from comparing herself to others.

I am so excited to anticipate how this book helps Sandy and all the women like us, who compare ourselves to others and judge ourselves unfairly.

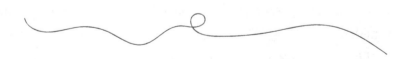

# Part Two

# "IT'S NOT A LEVEL PLAYING FIELD, I CAN'T COMPETE."

## CASE STUDY: CHEREE

Cheree, a bubbly seventy-two-year-old woman, came to see me for guidance.

*"I just want to look a bit better, that's all."*

*Cheree had a fabulous personality and a cheeky sense of humour.*

*"Nothing too drastic, I don't want anyone confusing me with my daughter. That would be awkward at family functions, wouldn't it?!" Cheree said with a glint in her eye.*

*Cheree had beautiful cheeks that mirrored her personality.*

*"Your cheeks are your Unique Facial Feature, so we must make the areas around your cheeks fade away into the background rather than take the focus from your cheeks."*

I explained the lead and supporting actor analogy to Cheree. As she was a retired professional dancer, it made perfect sense to her.

Cheree had a realistic body image and understood the limitations in what we could achieve in the clinic. She wanted to look good for her age. Cheree was also conscious of looking natural and was worried about looking over-treated. She had come to me on the suggestion of a friend who she felt looked, "so natural and fresh, almost like she's had nothing done."

We discussed a long-term plan for Cheree. We agreed on small incremental treatments that would be "just enough" to keep her looking fresh and feeling good, but not enough for anyone to notice. Small amounts of dermal filler placed in the areas of Cheree's lower face to support the tissue and reduce any shadowing. Small quantities of Botox to soften the negative emotion lines in her frown and forehead. Even smaller amounts of Botox to minimise the pull-down of the muscles that create the mouth frown. Little bits here, little bits there.

*"I have a friend who's had too much done," Cheree confided. "She's my closest friend, and we meet every week for coffee. I think she looks strange, but I would never tell her that, of course."*

*"Of course," I said.*

*"But she looks so good in photos. I don't get it. Every time we meet, she takes a photo of us and puts it on her Facebook page. I'm not a big Facebook user, but she tags me in the photos, and she looks great in them. I, on the other hand, look awful. That's why I'm here."*

I sensed her friend was a motivating factor in why Cheree was seeing me, so I allowed her to discuss it as she wanted to. Often women mention a 'friend' or someone they know who looks over-treated and who they want to avoid resembling. It gives them a chance to get reassurance from me that I won't make them look over-treated.

Cheree saw her friend every week and couldn't understand how in person she looked, "over-treated" and "strange," but the effect didn't translate in the photos she posted.

*"The problem is, when she puts these photos of the two of us up, everyone always makes comments complimenting her on how great she looks. It affects me. I know it shouldn't, it's silly really, I know I'm seventy-two for goodness' sake, but I still want to look good. I'm still a woman."*

---

I understand females of all ages want to look good and we gauge our appearance on those around us. We compare ourselves to them. How they look to us and how they look to others. Rarely do women know what their Unique Facial Feature is, so they rarely consider how what's beautiful about them differs from what is attractive about their friends.

---

"I even had a friend of ours call me and ask me if I was all right because I looked so bad compared to my friend in one photo that she put up on her Facebook page."

Cheree had been feeling so self-conscious about these photos her friend insisted on taking weekly, she started to look pretty miserable in them. She dreaded them.

*"I asked her why we had to take photos every week, and she said she wanted to have the memory. I told her she's so much more photogenic than me, and she just shrugged. I don't think she noticed how bad I looked in the photos she took."*

*Cheree put it down to her not being photogenic, but she still couldn't work out why her friend looked over-treated in the flesh, but great in the photos she took every week.*

## You can't choose facial features like deciding on ingredients to put in your smoothie.

It's not fair when only lips, or only cheeks, or foreheads are posted on social media to advertise cosmetic injectables. It's why I seldom post before and after pictures. It creates the idea that you can choose facial features like deciding on ingredients to put in your smoothie.

If you want to buy a handbag, you want to see the whole thing, not just the straps or the buckle. The buckle might look great, and you probably could imagine having that buckle on a handbag you already have. But you want to see the whole handbag so you can see if you like it or not.

It's hard to have willing participants who aren't in their 20s, who'll happily let before-and-after photos of their whole face be displayed on social media. Sometimes the only way a patient will consent to having their photo posted is if we promise to show their facial features in isolation. I've been guilty of showing single facial features, and I've contributed to the idea that individual features can be bought in isolation when they can't. Often, they won't suit your face. It's why I rarely post before-and-after photos on my social media pages that aren't of a whole face.

You met Nessie in Chapter Two. Nessie's self-proclaimed addiction to taking screenshots of other women was in the hope she'd put together a menu of ideal features for her face. It's not a level playing field when facial features are broken down individually and displayed by clinics on social media. And, unless the account holder admits they've used filters and face tuning apps, it's downright cruel to post edited photos.

I've seen this tactic used multiple times by celebrities. No one wants to call out people who feel the need to post heavily filtered photos of themselves. If someone feels the need to do this, they're hiding a lack of self-worth and don't think they're good enough as they are.

I believe when that person has a following of girls and women who look up to them; they have a responsibility to be truthful and honest with their audience. In posting filtered photos of themselves, they tell us we're not good enough unless we look like a perfected version of ourselves. I'm not talking about tweaking lighting. I am talking about making their nose smaller, lips and eyes bigger, eyebrows more arched, chin smaller, body thinner, breasts and bottom bigger and perkier. You name it, now there's an app that can do it all. Thankfully Instagram accounts whose sole purpose is to expose celebrities who post filtered images, is attempting to restore balance, but we need to recognise ourselves, when we're being fooled.

It started with airbrushing in magazines and has escalated to the point where anyone can be an editor and tweak their photos. I've witnessed friends and acquaintances do it and then reap the rewards of praise from people.

The small hit of dopamine they get from the positive comments is lovely, for sure, but it's not lasting and a mere Band-aid to what's eating them up. Their mirror doesn't lie. They feel worse because, not only is the thing they're trying to hide staring them straight back in the face, but the mirror is calling them out for lying.

## How to avoid the PUF train.

- Consider why you want to have cosmetic injections done in the first place and then each time after that. It will ensure you have realistic expectations of what cosmetic injections can do for you.
- Learn how to recognise and, therefore, beautify your very own Unique Facial Feature. Sadly, few practitioners know how to identify your Unique Facial Feature, let alone enhance it with cosmetic injectables. Arming yourself with the knowledge allows you to avoid having treatments done just because everyone else is doing them.
- Stop trying to heal something within you by getting stuff injected into your face, and
- Meet your Peeps.

CHEREE CONTINUED.

## Something fishy is going on...

*"One week we met with our other friend, the lady who recommend me to see you. Again, my friend took her photo, but of all three of us this time. She posted it as usual, on her Facebook page. This time, both my friend and I looked pretty awful, yet my friend looked great. She was standing in the middle, and someone commented 'Rose between two thorns.' That hurt me. I called our other friend, and I asked her why we looked awful. I mean, my friend looks fantastic in real life, I saw it with my own eyes, but even she looked ugly in these photos. I asked my friend if we might have both been unphotogenic. You'll never believe what she said."*

*I had my suspicions.*

*"That our friend was using a face fixing program she has on her phone to make her look prettier."*

*Cheree hadn't heard of this before, and so on the phone the other friend gave her a quick run-down on what it was.*

*"I was shocked. All this time, I've felt miserable about how I look in comparison to her, and she's been fooling us. I was hurt."*

It's so tricky when it's not a level playing field out there. When social media has everyone fooled, and you compare yourself to something that isn't even true. It's difficult enough when selfies are edited, but especially when there is more than one person in the photo, you are in the photos with them, and they've 'fixed' their face.

*"On the phone I told the other friend how I felt like I wasn't good enough. I told her that she was ageing beautifully. That's when she told me about you. I want to look as good as her."*

We completed Cheree's treatment and she returned one month later for the next phase of her treatment.

*She looked great. I was happy with how natural and soft her face looked. Her Unique Facial Feature was now lighting up her face. The areas of volume loss in her lower face no longer noticeable.*

*"I know I look better. I feel better because of it, too, but I wish I could pull this back some more, though."*

*Cheree grabbed at the skin on the sides of her cheeks and pulled it back. It often happens after the first treatment. Women look better and feel better, and then they want more, a more significant effect. It's easy to spiral down the rabbit hole of seeking perfection. I wondered what changed for Cheree.*

*"How's your friend?" I asked.*

*"I'm still meeting her every week. She commented that I looked well the other day, which she's never done before, so I must look better."*

*"Is she still posting the photos of you both?"*

*"Yes, and still doing the face editing thing. I haven't said anything about knowing what she's doing. Now I know about it, it annoys me, but I try to ignore it."*

*All the while Cheree is examining her face closely in the mirror and pulling and lifting at bits of her face.*

*"We have an excellent plan for you Cheree, let's stick to it. We are doing slow and steady things to restore your facial balance and keep your cheeks as your Unique Facial Feature."*

*"I know. I am realistic; I am. I don't want to look over-treated like my friend does in real life."*

*"Have you considered un-tagging yourself from your friend's photos?"*

*"No, I wouldn't know how to, but have started to take my own photos of us together and am putting these up on my Facebook page. No filter, no nothing. It's my way of being truthful, so that other women out there don't feel awful like I did."*

*I nodded in agreement.*

*Cheree giggled, "You'd think at our age, we'd be over this stuff, hey? But it goes on forever."*

Cheree understood, although she could be easily tempted into wanting more done to her face, she would never achieve the look of a photoshopped picture. She knew how to remain rational.

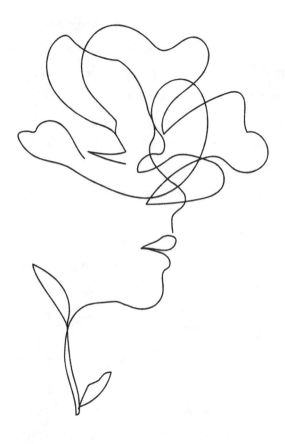

# Chapter Five

## Part One

# 'NO' IS NOT A DIRTY WORD.

CASE STUDY: ANNIE

The appointment note read, 'wants lips done.' I saw my new patient, Annie, in the waiting room and was immediately worried for her (and me). I knew this appointment and every subsequent one after, if she stayed with me, would be challenging.

Annie's lips were already overfilled and bizarre-looking, like those you see on some reality TV contestants. As I walked closer to her, I could also see her cheeks were too big for her petite face, and her tear troughs had been so severely overfilled, her eyes look abnormally small. It's a generalisation, but people who say to my reception staff when booking an appointment that they "want their lips done," aren't familiar with their Unique Facial Feature. I invited Annie into my treatment room and took a deep breath in to ground me.

Annie was twenty-six years old, so young. A successful finance entrepreneur. The first thing she said to me was, "Money is no object. I have all the money I need for whatever you think I'll need."

Going by how much dermal filler was already in Annie's face, many of the practitioners who'd treated her in the past, had taken advantage of her generosity. They'd seen this as an opportunity to make money from a vulnerable young woman. They'd swallowed their ethical and moral compass and started filling her poor little face up.

Sadly, Annie thought that by declaring that money was no object, she'd receive the very best of care.

*"I've been watching you for a while, but thought that you couldn't be that good because you aren't located in the city and you don't have thousands of followers."*

Although Annie lived only twenty minutes away from my clinic, for the previous two years, she'd driven past my clinic to attend the 'big fancy ones' in the city. She was under the illusion city clinics would be better. A common assumption to make.

*"I've been to five different clinics over the last eighteen months, and I still don't look any better,"* Annie said.

*"Why did you choose to go to those clinics?"* I asked.

*"They're heavily promoted on Instagram by all the influencers. I thought I'd look like them if I went there, too."*

And there it was, another intelligent and sassy young woman sucked in by the influencer advertising.

*"Annie, the influencers don't even look like they do on their Instagram pages,"* I said.

*"I know. I can't believe I was so stupid,"* Annie replied.

*"You're far from stupid, Annie. You're brave and smart to have seen through it and make the change. I'll look after you, but I'll also be honest with you and tell you what you do and don't need to have done to your face. Are you ok with that?" I asked.*

*"I think so," she said.*

I examined Annie's face, which took some doing. It was tough to establish what was natural to her and what had been injected. I asked her what treatments she'd had done. She remembered some, but not all.

*"I don't know what they do when I'm in there."*

I hear this comment a lot. Sadly, people don't know what treatments they've had. With Annie, it was a guessing game, but by looking and feeling her face, I jogged her memory about possible treatments she had received in the past.

I noted a rather sizeable sausage-like bulge in her right temple area. It had a bluish tinge to it.

*"Have you had dermal filler in your temple area?" I asked.*

*"Yes, I have. I forgot about that. About three months ago, I had someone inject me there. I think it's a bit swollen still. It hurt when he injected the right side. And it's often painful still. I get pain in my forehead and headaches since the treatment too," Annie said.*

*"Did you contact the clinic?" I asked.*

*"No, I didn't bother. I didn't want to go back again. I was in there for a total of ten minutes and I spent $3000. He didn't examine my face at all, just started putting the needles in, until he injected my temple, and I cried out in pain. He wasn't very nice to me and practically pushed me out of the room after that," she said.*

I noted a hardened trail extending from Annie's temple up to her forehead area. I explained that dermal filler placed incorrectly can be dangerous and asked her if she was happy for me to dissolve the filler in her right temple.

*"I was going to ask you if I could have more dermal filler there, actually." She pointed to her forehead and right temple area. "I look flat through here."*

I explained to Annie that she didn't have a flat temple, but the bulge made the surrounding area look sunken. I promised we'd restore it to looking less sunken this way. She was happy for me to dissolve the whole area around her temple and forehead. Within minutes of doing so, the hardness softened, and Annie said the aching reduced.

Here was a young woman who was a ticking time bomb. I can't imagine what would've happened if she'd had more filler injected into her temple area as she'd wanted. But Annie was developing trust in me. She told me she wanted her lips refilled. A classic sign of body dysmorphia is being unable to see the areas of your face that are already overfilled. And always hunting for more in the hope it will give you a look you desire.

When we separate each facial feature, we end up chasing what we feel are perfect facial features—lips like this, cheeks like that, a jaw like this one, and so on. When we chase perfect features, our risk of becoming a weird over-treated face goes through the roof. We'll never achieve the look we're striving to achieve.

Our facial features are not in isolation from the rest of our face. You must be able to identify your Unique Facial Feature. Better still, have a practitioner who can identify it for you. Then, you can create treatment plans that aim to highlight your Unique Facial Feature and enhance a beautiful and unique face.

Sadly, Annie's face was completely unbalanced. Her face was so out of proportion that she looked unusual. Annie's naturally pretty face no longer appeared as pretty as it should.

## "I'm twenty-six years old and he thought I was fifty."

At only twenty-six years of age, Annie looked much older.

*"Everyone thinks I am older than I am. They think I am in my late 50s. It's depressing. I'm single, and a guy I met last week at a work function asked if I'd had my big birthday yet. I thought he meant my 21st, and I said yes, but he meant my 50th! I left a few minutes later. I told him I'd forgotten to turn my iron off and practically ran out of the bar,"* Annie said.

Too much and poorly placed dermal fillers and Botox make you look older than you are. I've already covered the reasons in chapter one of this book. But as a quick refresher:

When young women get too much done to their faces, they lose that ability to express emotions. The marker that tells us how plump and youthful their skin is by bouncing back after expressing the emotion, gets removed. Second, it's considered an anti-ageing treatment. The assumption that only older women get treatment convinces people you must therefore be older if you have an overfilled and over-frozen face. At least middle-aged or beyond.

One thing's for sure, overfilled faces **always** look older than they are. I haven't done the double-blind, randomised, placebo-controlled study to prove it. Still, I have my own experiences and those of other people I've spoken to confirm my theory.

In writing this book, I pondered on and explored why this is so. Why do women look so much older? Is it because, as mentioned in chapter one, they have no emotion? Is it because it's so apparent that the extra volume in their lips, cheeks, jaw, chin, tear troughs and so on, isn't real, therefore they must be older? What is it?

I remember watching 'Housewives of Melbourne' and being

stunned at learning the age of one woman. I assumed from her face she was in her late 50s or early 60s, but in fact, she was in her early 40s. It was shocking. She looked so much older because she'd overfilled her face and was completely frozen. Void of any emotion, it was impossible to tell what she was feeling and thinking. The only way we knew what she was feeling, and thinking was by what she said. Even then, it was hard to gauge whether she was being serious or joking because the small nuances we show when displaying emotion were completely gone. Even to my trained eye, her appearance fooled me. So, it's not surprising that the untrained eye gets it wrong.

This doesn't make sense, does it? When the reason we get work done is to make us look younger. When we get the right amount of work done, and it highlights our Unique Facial Feature, we do look younger, fresher, softer, and happier. But when we get too much work done, we look older. ALWAYS. When Annie commented, everyone thought she looked older than twenty-six, I understood. Of course, she looked older. Her face was overfilled and over-frozen.

ANNIE CONTINUED.

After dissolving the dermal filler that sat dangerously in the vessel that fed blood to her forehead and right temple, I got to work at reversing the damage done over the last two years.

Annie's was a tricky case. But I felt confident that, by understanding her face and her personality, I could transform her from being an overfilled and over-frozen face, back to be the beautiful young woman she was.

*"Can I dissolve the dermal filler in your lips?" I asked.*

*"No," she replied.*

*Ok, so maybe this wouldn't be as straightforward as I hoped. Remember, Annie booked her first appointment with me with the instruction she "wants lips done." I needed to go gently with her.*

*"So, looking at your face Annie, your lips are large, and your chin is small. We need to rebalance your lower face so that what we see when we look at you, is not just your lips."*

*"Ok, but I don't want my lips smaller. They're already small."*

Annie genuinely believed her lips were small. They were much larger than any of my regular patients' lips. Patients with body dysmorphia will rarely let you dissolve any of the dermal fillers they already have in their faces. I'll always suggest dissolving to patients whose lips are overfilled.

I've had patients go elsewhere to have their lips filled because I refuse to put any more filler into them. They'll have the other areas of their face treated with me but go to whichever clinic is having a crazy special on lip filler and have their lips done there. When they come back to me for their next appointment, I'll immediately notice they've had their lips filled up again.

They hope they can get away with it and I won't notice, but there's nothing about a face that I won't remember. It generally goes like this:

*"Hello... It's so lovely to see you. You've had your lips done again, haven't you?"*

The look on their faces is often of shock.

*"I just got a little bit. They'd really gone down."*

*"I understand. How much did you get?"*

*"1ml (or 2ml, or 3ml)."*

*"Ok. Let's look at you and work on the rest of your face."*

It's all good and well having more and more injected into your lips. After all, we're all adults here and can make decisions for ourselves. And yes, if you look at each feature separately, then you will, of course, see your lips will deflate over time. They will flatten considerably in the first two weeks after having your lips injected because it was swelling, not lip filler that initially made them look so 'inflated'. Try not to get confused between what's swelling and what's dermal filler. They are two totally different things. The problem is, dermal filler can last for years and years in our faces and just like Annie discovered, the bigger your lips are, the more they protrude out and down. Not only is it the main and absurd feature of your face, but it dilutes your Unique Facial Feature and makes your other features look small, unbalanced and don't belong on your face. It then becomes a game of each feature trying to outdo the other. Like magic, a Pretty Ugly Face gets created.

Annie's lips were so big, I needed to fill and rebalance her chin considerably. Her chin was practically non-existent beneath her lips, which also made her look older. As we age, our chin gets smaller and lifts. I stood back, observed Annie's face from all sides, and was satisfied with the result of her treatment. I gave Annie the mirror, and luckily, she was happy too.

*"Does that mean you can do more in my lips?"*

*"No, Annie."*

It's a very delicate relationship between facial features and overall beauty. When I talk about enhancing the face, I talk about half a millimetre to one millimetre of change. Subtle and tiny modifications only. It's also a very delicate relationship between the body dysmorphic patient and their clinician.

In my first appointment with Annie, I needed to gain her trust, take her hand, and steer her away from the possibility of further hurt from being overfilled and over-frozen. Annie didn't know the extent to which she was physically and mentally damaged by the poor treatments she'd received. All she knew was the procedures she'd had done previously hadn't made her happy the way she hoped they would.

## How to stop being so greedy. Gluttony.

The Merriam-Webster Dictionary defines gluttony as 'habitual greed.' **https://www.merriam-webster.com/dictionary/glutton 11/6/2020**

Author Peter De Vries said, "Gluttony is an emotional escape, a sign something is eating us." **https://allauthor.com/ quotes/27925/ 11/6/2020**. Never have I read a more accurate description of society's disease.

When we look to external physical things to make us happy, there is something eating us up inside.

> Gluttony is very much a symptom of life today. See it, want it, buy it, have it. Want more, have more, more and more and more and more. And no need to wait!

Society has let us down. We have let ourselves down. The concern we have today is we're no longer content. Why should we be when told we can have anything we want? As women, this is truer than ever before in history. You'd like a high-powered career? Go for it, girl! You'd like to be an entrepreneur and run a successful business? Go for it, girl! *And* you'd like to have a family and be an incredible mum and partner? Go for it, girl! The pressure is immense.

As women, we should be allowed to have whatever we want. Absolutely. As young women, we're pretty good at achieving this. We want that Gucci handbag; we get it. We want that outfit; we get it. We want those bigger lips; we get them. If we want those lashes, those breasts, that chiselled jaw and plumped up cheeks; we get them. The women we follow on Instagram have all these things too, and they look happy and fulfilled. We want that too.

It's the never-ending desire to keep filling the bucket, rather than tending to the items we already have. Money is no concern because we can get whatever we want on credit cards, Afterpay, Zip Pay, and even payment plans with individual businesses. Before hitting our bank account, we can arrange for every last bit of our wage to be sent to multiple businesses to pay off multiple purchases we've made.

The idea of owning our own home has become so unattainable that saving for a home seems fruitless. The instant hit we feel from a purchase in-store or online is enough to give us a quick high. So many carrots dangled in front of us. Instagram, Snapchat, Facebook, Influencers and celebrity-endorsed products and services that we 'cannot live without.' Why should you miss out? Remember, fear sells.

## Get out of bed, girl, get hustling!!

We're encouraged to get as much out of our day as possible. Wake earlier than anyone else. Those who snooze, lose, but not us. If only we go to bed later and wake earlier, we can beat the competition. Fit more into our day, our week, our month, and our year. Break down our day into tasks, better still, break it into twenty-five-minute slots, and have a task allocated for each of those slots. Get the stuff done. If we don't, someone else will, and we'll stay at the bottom of the heap—a loser. Compete with others, compete with ourselves.

It's the same with cosmetic procedures. I have met women who are still paying off the breast augmentations and rhinoplasties they had five years ago. Some have even been paying off the first breast augmentation when they need to go in for the next one, ten years later.

Budgeting and allocating money for personal upkeep is essential. Today we see women (and men, but this book is for women), overextending themselves. Before I started writing this book, the Therapeutic Goods Administration (TGA) of Australia changed the law to permit finance options like Zip Pay and Afterpay for the payment of cosmetic medicine services. Previously, the TGA believed these 'on credit' payment methods unethically lured patients who otherwise couldn't afford to have the medical procedure done.

Our brains and bodies clutter with constantly updated information, tasks that we must achieve, and things we must have. We are hoarders of things we hope will make us happy.

## Shrink your brain.

When we sleep, our brain shrinks by 20%. Like a sponge, our brain shrinks, squeezing the waste from it. The liquid waste then travels down our spinal cord, and fresh cerebral spinal fluid removes the toxins, and new nutrient rich fluid moves in waves back up to the brain. We are the most intelligent creatures, aren't we?! I'm so in love with the human body and its processes. Like our Peeps, our physical body has one aim in our lives, to keep us regulated, happy, and safe. When our brain is too cluttered, the sponge struggles to contract and squeeze out the waste. Thereby the effects of chronic stress have commenced.

Chronic stress today comes from the continual belief that we're not enough. We need to achieve more. Fear of Missing Out (FOMO) is a relatively new phenomenon, only sixteen years old. Describing what happens when we believe others have better experiences than us. No one likes to miss out. We learn quickly as children when sweets get handed out. The world comes crashing down if we get less.

Social Media platforms allow our FOMO to operate at consistently high levels. A study described in Sherry Turkle's book 'Alone Together.' **https://www.theguardian.com/books/2011/ jan/30/alone-together-sherry-turkle-review 20/05/2020**

The article describes a twenty-eight-year-old woman and successful advertising executive who lived in a shared house with other professionals. She felt fine about her life until she opened Facebook and saw a post by a friend. The post showed a picture of her friend, with her husband and their new baby in their new home. Suddenly the woman felt like she 'wanted to die.' In retaliation, the woman trawled through photos from her weekend, picked the one showing her having the 'most fun', and posted it with a comment about how 'awesome' her life was. However, she didn't believe a word of it. Undoubtedly, another person saw her post and felt FOMO, too. And, so, the cycle continues.

Fear stunts our physical growth as children. It also stunts our physical and mental growth as adults. Fear of Missing Out. The belief other people *know* the secret to look beautiful, and no one has told you about it, creates chronic stress amongst women of all ages. Social media plays into the hands of FOMO and forces us always to compare ourselves to other women.

At the height of my stress-induced burnout, I would wake at 2am with a massive rush of cortisol. It would jolt me with a start. It signalled the beginning of my day. I immediately fretted over the things I needed to do, and immediately I'd predict I wouldn't achieve all the stuff I needed to. I'd get the shakes and feel like I was running a race. My poor brain and body should've been rejuvenating and healing. Yet, I'd be awake imagining the worst-case scenario of every possible thing in my life. Catastrophising if you will. Then, at about 6 am when I was due to wake, convinced of my failings as a mother and wife, my body racked with exhaustion; I'd fall asleep to my sobbing.

But we don't need to have it all. We don't need to *be* it all.


ANNIE CONTINUED.
Annie returned three months later and then three months after that. Even though she met a partner and moved away for his career, she still returned to me every three months. At every appointment, Annie asked me to treat her lips and temples and put more in her cheeks. Each time she let me nurture and educate her on why it was important to continue to highlight her Unique Facial Feature, which was her eyes. By the end of that first year together, Annie

thanked me for helping her and never taking advantage of her vulnerability as others had done before. She told me that for the first time ever, people had commented on how beautiful she was looking.

The challenge of keeping Annie off of the slippery slope to PUFdom was constant. At every appointment, because I was not permitted to dissolve the filler in her lips, I had to build up her lower face to balance her features.

Annie has not been unfaithful to me. She hasn't seen another aesthetic medicine practitioner while she's been in my care. She's not been taken advantage of again. I'm so proud of Annie. She's been so brave and, unlike many who are inundated with social media's continual pressure to 'have all the stuff' and look a certain way, she has trusted our process.

However, because Annie had so much dermal filler injected into her lips over the years, so much remains in there and may well last for years to come. This is why dissolving it would be the only way to know what her lips look like naturally. Even then, because her lips were distended with so much dermal filler, they'd likely look very deflated. At every appointment, I asked Annie if I could dissolve her lip filler, even just a small amount. Every time she refused and would recoil. I could see she felt hurt by my continued attempts. I must always tread lightly.

We always did very mild and subtle treatments with Annie. I got excited every time I finished treating her. I handed her the mirror knowing I had kept her safe from looking like an overfilled and over-frozen face for the time being. And she looked beautiful and unique when she left my clinic. A little less PUF and a little more normal. But even then, once she left, the battle was hers to fight. She needed to trust her Unique Facial Feature, her Peeps,

Tapping, and Mantra to keep her safe. Safe from herself and the pressures everyone feels today. It's a constant battle. I could lead her to water, but I could not make her drink. I could educate her. And, while she understood what I was saying when she was with me, I couldn't be on her shoulder each time she got sucked into the self-loathing and comparison rabbit hole that comes with social media.

The last time I saw Annie and handed her the mirror to examine our work, she looked closely at her face in the mirror and said:

*"Should I get plastic surgery for these little wrinkles beneath my eyes?"*

It's like an alcoholic who cannot have even one small drink after becoming teetotal. Body dysmorphic patients will never live up to the expectations they have of themselves.

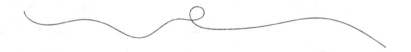

## Part Two

# DECLUTTER YOUR FACE.

I don't know about you, but when I'm feeling overwhelmed, I like to declutter. I know that since Marie Kondo, it's become a buzzword, but show me any rabbit hole mindset that doesn't improve with a good old dose of decluttering. It might be our bedroom, our clothes, the people we follow on social media, or our mindset. Accompanied by a lovely round of chatting to our Peeps, Tapping it out, and saying our Mantra, decluttering works a treat. Once decluttered, we can step away from the space or mindset and breathe a sigh of relief at the beauty that we've uncovered.

I believe it's the same with our faces. A good old dose of facial decluttering is hugely cathartic and ensures what remains is all that's important. Guess what that is? Absolutely! Our Unique Facial Feature is all that remains when we declutter our face.

Decluttering is a prime way of ensuring we don't become gluttonous. It's so easy to get sucked into the trap of having it all by considering our facial features separately. I must have the perfect jaw, the perfect lips, the perfect chin, the perfect cheeks, the perfect nose, the perfect wrinkle-free face. Still, we know that having too many incredible paintings on one wall means none of them stand out. None of their beauty is apparent. In this case, we are decluttering our face, quietly confident that we are showcasing our unique facial feature and our most beautiful and unique face.

> Knowing and trusting in the power of your Unique Facial Feature, and remembering the anchors you've so bravely established, will reduce your chances of becoming gluttonous.

I recently presented at a cosmetic medicine conference for fellow practitioners. I shared the message of this book about how we're losing our beauty and becoming uglier thanks to our obsession with *having it all*. See it, want it, buy it, have it. I shared my experience of the social epidemic that we can and must have it all! That we must perfect every single facial feature.

My presentation aimed to empower my audience - Providing them with the knowledge and strength to say 'no' if they believed that a patient was getting sucked into the modern disease of needing to have it all. The audience not only got it, but they started implementing my techniques immediately in their clinics. One audience member sent me a message. She told me that, since hearing my presentation, she finally felt strong enough to educate and nurture patients who she worried were becoming lost in the obsession of perfecting every facial feature.

If I can empower practitioners as much as the general public about how to fall in love with Beautiful Unique Faces, we're getting everyone on the same side. The side of unique beauty, the side against perfection.

# Learning to say NO.

There are thousands of wonderful practitioners out there. Those of us who care deeply for our patients still find one part of our role incredibly challenging—the ability to say 'No.' I regularly say 'No' if it's what my patient needs to hear. When we say 'No' to our patients, the vast majority accept our reasoning and are grateful for our honesty and care for them.

Of all the thousands of people I've treated throughout my career, I've only asked two people to seek treatment elsewhere. They were both hugely empowering moments for me. No longer could I assist either of these patients and, quite frankly, they'd both become nasty. Their inability to practice restraint and respect for their face filtered through into disrespect of me. They had fixated ideas on what they could command of me and my team. The treatments they demanded were not in their best interest and I'd felt increasingly uncomfortable every time I said, 'No.' to each of them.

Redirecting away from 'having it all, more is better' mindset to educate and nurture women back to a healthier outlook on their beautiful unique face is my stance. Sometimes patients cross the boundaries of a professional relationship and become abusive. People become angry and frustrated when they can't get their way. But it's our responsibility as clinicians to do what's best, even if our patients sometimes disagree. I ended these relationships and advised both patients to seek future treatment elsewhere. I respect anyone who on seeing a relationship isn't working, leaves that relationship.

## CASE STUDY: OLIVIA

Olivia was a thirty-seven-year-old senior executive. She saw an article I'd written on the benefits of prescription Vitamin A for acne sufferers. She was at the end of her tether with seeking help for her chronic skin condition.

Olivia consulted various skin salons and her general practice clinic for help with her acne. She'd been recommended and received facials, different skincare creams, and oral antibiotics for her acne. Nothing worked, and her acne was impacting both her physical and psychological health. She'd never received any cosmetic injectable treatments.

At our first appointment, Olivia was very depressed and frustrated with the state of her skin and the lack of help. She lived over two hours away from my clinic but was hopeful that I might help.

*"You're my last resort. I don't know what I will do if you can't help me."*

* No pressure for this high achieving people pleaser then.


Olivia had a combination of active acne and scarring present. Her acne was so severe it was creating more scarring. Once our skin becomes scarred, it is challenging to take the skin back to being smooth. Acne that causes scarring is considered an urgent medical condition and is classified the same as some of the most severe skin conditions. The damage can impact not only a person's face, but also their mental health. And means a patient with this type of acne is to be treated by a dermatologist immediately.

*"Have you been referred to a dermatologist by your GP?"*

*"No, my GP has had me on antibiotics for twelve months. So far they haven't made any difference to my skin."*

Doctors had diagnosed Olivia with endometriosis and polycystic ovary syndrome. Both of which can contribute to and cause adult acne in women. She'd been taking the oral contraceptive pill for the previous two years, which is a valid treatment for women with acne.

I promised her we'd do all we could to help treat her acne. Because she came from a profession that valued procedure and protocol highly, I broke Olivia's treatment plan into clear cut and measurable steps for her.

*"Olivia, I understand how your skin is affecting your self-esteem. It's painful, and you hate the way it looks. It's not fair, is it, that you have this condition? You just want to feel and look better. I know. You have cystic acne, which I regard as a serious medical condition. Today, I'll start you on two medicated skin creams that will help to treat the infection and inflammation of your skin and another that will increase your skin's cell turnover. Meaning the pilosebaceous unit (or the hair and oil gland of your skin) will have a chance to normalise. Your pilosebaceous unit isn't functioning as best it could, which is causing your acne," I explained.*

*"I will give you a form today that you can take as soon as possible to get a blood sample collected. I will ask for the blood results to go to the dermatologist who I am going to refer you to. I would like you to call them today and request an urgent appointment. You will tell them you have been diagnosed with severe cystic acne with significant scarring to your face. I'll call the dermatologist's rooms also and request you're seen urgently. Normal waiting time of six months should be reduced to approximately four weeks if we both do this. Although your skin may show some signs of improvement with the skin creams*

*I'm prescribing you; I believe you need a medication called Isotretinoin, the tablet form of one of the creams I'm giving you. You can expect to be on Isotretinoin tablets for six to nine months. The dermatologist will keep me informed of your progress. Once you start these tablets, you'll stop using the creams you're starting on today, but given it will likely be four weeks until you see the dermatologist, we must start treating it right away."*

*Olivia, who'd been nodding in agreement throughout my explanation of her plan, started to cry.*

*"I've lost faith in anyone being able to help me, but I think this might work."*

*I placed my hand on Olivia's arm. "I will help you through this, anyway I can. Have you got any acne on your body?"*

*At this point, Olivia's cries turned into sobs. She couldn't answer but lifted her top to show her acne covered back and chest. Then she rolled her sleeves up to show me her arms and rolled her trouser legs up to show me her calves. Olivia had the same acne and scarring all over her body.*

*"I always have to wear clothes that cover my arms, legs, chest. The anxiety I experience getting dressed..."*

Regardless of the weather, Olivia wore long sleeves to cover her arms, and long pants or skirts to cover her legs. Social functions presented a different kind of concern. Olivia would either make excuses not to attend or would hide her body under elaborate clothing. She wore similar style clothing for work and play.

Olivia also picked at the scarring that remained when the cysts got better. She knew where each scar was and could tell me how many days she'd been picking at that one. She felt a sense of control over her skin condition with knowing how long that particular scar had been there and how many times she'd picked at it that day. The satisfaction she felt, from feeling the roughened skin from the scarring turn smooth, after she had picked it, gave her a false sense of comfort. Olivia's skin condition was having a significant impact on her mental health and, at various times during our consultation, she was inconsolable.

*"Can I get some Botox in my frown and forehead, too?"*

*We hadn't discussed any other treatments. Olivia's comment caught me off guard. I hadn't noticed her frown and forehead wrinkles, only her acne.*

*"Do you mind if we wait until you have seen the dermatologist and have seen an improvement in your acne?"*

*Olivia was happy to wait.*

She saw the dermatologist who agreed she needed to be started on Isotretinoin ASAP for her skin and mental health. She was medicated on Isotretinoin for ten months with a break of two months in the middle of that time.

Two months after Olivia started care under the dermatologist, she came in to see me again. Her skin showed signs of improvement, and she was feeling better.

*"It's incredible. I have patches of clear skin now."*

*She showed me a small area on her chest and forehead that had no active cysts.*

*"I haven't had this much clear skin for years."*

*"Oh, Olivia, that is wonderful. I'm so happy for you."*

*"I'm concerned with my frown lines. They make me look angry. I used to be so focused on my acne that, even though I could see my angry frown lines, they didn't bother me so much. Now I can see them because my skin is clearing up and looking so much better."*

*I could see Olivia's static frown and forehead lines now, too.*

*"I feel old and drawn and tired. It's been a hard few years, and I feel like my face is showing it."*

*I asked Olivia to frown and create some other facial movements.*

*"It's weird. People who've never said anything before are asking me if I'm ok. One of my team told a colleague that he hadn't wanted to ask for time off to take his wife to chemotherapy because I looked so angry. I mean, that's bad, isn't it? This poor guy needs to be with his wife, and he's too scared even to approach me because I look like I'm about to bite his head off."*

I discussed the options for Olivia to help improve the appearance of the lines in the negative areas (frown, forehead) on her face. I also discussed the movement and loss of fat pads in the face that contribute to the drawn, tired, and unhappy look she was complaining of.

I treated her with dermal filler. Injecting it into the areas of her face where volume restoration was required. I also injected a small amount of Botox into the various muscles of her face contributing to the appearance of negative emotions. Olivia was happy with the *immediate* changes she saw in the mirror from the dermal filler. She understood the muscle relaxant took two weeks to kick in.

*"Thank you so much. When I come here; I feel so much better about myself when I leave."*

Three months later and Olivia had been on Isotretinoin for five months. Her skin was clear, yet dry and flaky. These were expected side effects from her treatment. She coped with these side effects with regular emollients and occlusive moisturisers. Olivia was in good spirits. She was seeing the effects of medication. The angry and painful acne cysts on her face and body were clearing. Her scarring was less raised. She was working hard to stop picking the existing scars. Some, though, she continued to regularly re-open as though through the comfort of habit.

*"I'm not sure what I would do without these scars to pick."*

She picked in areas she could access without drawing attention to herself at work. She would wear dark-coloured tops to disguise the oozing blood spots that appeared on her clothing. The medication makes skin fragile. While her skin was improving remarkably, her hidden skin was suffering more permanent scarring from her continued picking. Olivia cried as she lifted her top to show me the trauma she was inflicting on herself. Picking was a way Olivia had learned to release the brain's chemical endorphin. She would scan her skin for hardened lumps and bumps of sores, pick them, and then enjoy the resulting smoothness of her skin.

Together, we discussed other ways Olivia could feel the satisfaction she got from picking a scab off, from different, healthier habits. Olivia was open to the idea. She was embarrassed about what she was doing to herself. We used Olivia's wedding ring as a substitute. She could touch that. Feel the texture of it. Feel the width of it and the sensation of swivelling it around her finger. By taking mental note of how it felt while she touched it, she could be fully present. She got the same endorphin release as when picking a scab and feeling the smoothness of her skin beneath it, once the scab went.

Olivia is a high achiever. She made decisions quickly based on her extensive management skills and experience in risk aversion. Like many successful women today, Olivia had worked incredibly hard to build her career. Solution-focused, if there was a problem, she used her vast intellect and aptitude to devise solutions. It is what had seen her win awards and facilitated the rapid advancement of her career.

Olivia saw her adult acne as a problem that required medical intervention. Despite her attempts to solve the problem with visits to her GP, she couldn't get satisfactory answers or results. Hence, after reading the piece I'd written on acne, Olivia sought guidance from me. I explained why she was suffering from adult acne and, according to therapeutic guidelines, recommended the next best research-driven treatment option available to her. I could empathise with Olivia and reassured her that I agreed with her this was a problem that needed to be solved. I developed a plan with her to treat her acne, and we agreed on a system to assess the plan's effectiveness throughout the treatment process. Mostly, I too have a problem-solving focus and am process-driven.

One year after I'd first consulted Olivia, her dermatologist ceased her medication. Her skin was now completely clear of acne. It was a victory. Together we created a treatment plan that addressed her residual acne scarring and the areas of concern she had regarding her facial ageing. Olivia was nearing forty and, with her skin no longer covered in acne, she could see the effects growing up in North Queensland had on her skin.

During the next three years, which coincided with Olivia's rapid career advancements, I noticed she was becoming more obsessed with her appearance.

*"I look in the mirror a lot. I feel I can always find something wrong with my face. It's almost comforting to look in the mirror and find a fault. It grounds me. I can then start researching the solutions to the problems, which makes me feel like I'm in control," Olivia said.*

## Ageing is not a problem we can solve.

I've seen this in so many women over the years. However, ageing is not something we can ever have ultimate control over. We are human beings with a life cycle. As parts of our cells and tissue die, others are regenerating. Yes, there are certain choices we can make that will help our body to restore and age more slowly, but in the end, without wanting to sound morose, death comes to all of us.

## No one hates us more than we hate ourselves.

There is no 100% success rate with anti-ageing. You can't solve the problem entirely, so that there are no signs of ageing left at all. You can't defy ageing. It's the *'fighting ageing'* mindset that's seeing women globally becoming depressed, anxious, and exhausted. Our self-loathing for our face and body is off the Richter scale. No one hates us more than we hate ourselves. *That* is what needs to change.

---

*"I love my mummy, I love my daddy, I love my sister, and I love myself!"*

My daughters, who are six and eight years old, love themselves unconditionally. It's wonderful. When does this change, and why? I see the empowerment they feel when they say it. Their little lady bodies straighten up and grow strong. A knowing smile breaking on their lips. It's one of my favourite things to watch my daughters do.

---

From my experience in this profession, I believe it's getting worse. Not only is comparison the killer of creativity, but it's also the killer of self-care and love. Looking on social media at unhealthy examples of people who are 1-2 steps ahead of us and believing the stories they tell us. Comparing our face to their face. Our body to their body. Our career to their career. Constant comparison is killing us, ignoring our Peeps, binding our Tapping fingers, silencing our Mantras and making us the most miserable we've ever been.

## OLIVIA CONTINUED.

Olivia continued having maintenance treatments with me, but it was evident she was becoming frustrated with the limitations of non-surgical cosmetic medicine. At the peak of her frustration, it became apparent she believed I was to blame for her unhappiness. I couldn't reverse her facial ageing, remove her wrinkles, and completely smooth out her skin. Regardless of Olivia's intelligence and my attempt to continually educate her, she couldn't grasp the idea that her facial ageing was a problem that couldn't be solved.

Olivia sought treatment elsewhere and told me about it at her next appointment.

*"I booked into two other clinics, much closer to me and so much easier to get to."*

Olivia still travelled over two hours to reach my clinic. I understood her desire to find a closer practitioner.

*"As soon as I walked into each of these appointments, I felt sick in the stomach. Like I was being unfaithful to you. The people who consulted me were not you. They didn't consult me but instead offered me the package deals they had on sale. I knew more than they did, and that's because of what you'd taught me over the*

*years. I told them I didn't like my neck and my eyes. One of them suggested I have my frown treated, and the other said I needed lip fillers. I left both without having any treatment done."*

It was important for Olivia to see the grass wasn't necessarily greener on the other side, and she was happy to be back in my caring arms. We followed our original plan, tweaking it only when necessary, but doing all the things that brought us back to highlighting her Unique Facial Feature. Olivia was happy, and she was settled for about six months. After that, she started discussing the possibility of seeking surgical intervention for the things she didn't like about her face. Convinced her neck was saggier and under-eye area wrinklier than other women her age, Olivia told me she'd arranged an appointment with a prominent plastic surgeon.

## Here we were again.

Olivia was desperate to find solutions to her problems and an inability to accept anything less than a 100% correction. I confidently told her the surgeon would turn her away and suggest she revisit him in five years.

Olivia returned three months later. I was delighted to see her in my reception area. She hadn't had surgery and looked 'normal.'

*"I saw the surgeon." She said.*

*"Oh, great. How was that?" I asked.*

*"Yes, really good. He said I needed a facelift, liposuction, and upper and lower blepharoplasty, which is weird because I hadn't noticed how saggy my eyelids were until he showed me. He also said if I had all that, he'd do a full-thickness laser resurfacing treatment for half the normal price."*

*Aghast, I was silent.*

*Olivia looked at me as if to say, 'I told you so!'*

*I understood her being annoyed with me. I was annoyed with myself. A prominent plastic surgeon told her she needed surgery, in fact, multiple surgeries. And yet I'd told her she didn't need surgery. As far as she was concerned, I was not taking her concerns and fears about her face seriously. This guy had, though. He saw there were multiple things she'd be willing to have done, so he used the 'all or nothing' mindset. "You'll be under anaesthetic anyway; you may as well have it all done."*

*"What will you do?" I asked her.*

*"I would have had it done it already, but I was so busy last month with a work conference and couldn't take time off. I've booked in for the surgeries for next month. I've paid my deposit."*

*"What would you like to do today, Olivia?"*

*"Just my Botox, please."*

*I treated Olivia with her regular small maintenance doses. Neither of us spoke. I couldn't. I needed some time out to digest what the surgeon said to her and Olivia, well, she'd lost all faith in me now.*

*"I wish you could treat these lines under my eyes."*

*"Yes, it is indeed a tricky area. We cannot safely do dermal filler there, and if we spread the Botox under there too much, your lower eyelid will become saggy."*

*"Yes, I know. You've already told me that."*

*"PRP or threads are the best treatments for that area that I can do. It's safe to do PRP here because it is a risky area, plus it uses the natural healing and collagen-stimulating properties of your blood."*

*"I had that treatment a year ago, and it didn't work. Not even a little bit. I was very disappointed."*

With that, Olivia got off the treatment bed and left my room.

She did not rebook to see me again. As I said goodbye to her and wished her well for the week, I knew that it would be the last time I saw her.

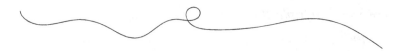

## Part Three

# EARN THE RIGHT TO SING.

You don't need to control everything.

Leave some mystery.

Perfection the number one enemy of happiness.

Olivia, Annie and Lucy are examples of how society tells us if we work harder, hustle more, grind when others are asleep, we can control every last bit of our lives. Beat our competitors, stand out from the crowd, set ourselves apart, make millions, and be the dictator of our lives.

I believe though, we can only control a tiny portion of our lives. What we eat, what we wear, and who we see, if we exercise, when we go to bed, what we think and how we think about ourselves and respond to others. We have little control over the most fundamental thing about us, though, our humanness. We can't control our cells. And we can't control our blood, our organs, our genes, our ageing process. The idea we can change and control everything has led us, I believe, into an epidemic of thinking we're not worthy as we are and must perfect the experience of being human. We're being conditioned into a sea of perfected control freaks and wearing it like a badge of honour. The more stress chemicals we produce in trying to control everything, the faster our bodies and faces fail us. Stressing and attempting to control every aspect of our lives, is counterproductive in our quest for beating ageing.

"I need to be in control." "I'm a control freak." "Everything must be perfect."

During my time at drama school, one of my mentors told me about the musical theatre principle of *'earning the right to sing.'* It described the moment the character happened upon their *'inciting incident.'* In literary terms, it describes a life-changing event that catapults the character into a new world or brand-new way of thinking.

My mentor described 'earning the right to sing' as being the ultimate release for the character and the audience. The moment when the tension was so electric the only way it could be released was through song. The character had no control over what was happening to them. The song's release meant they could work out what was holding them back and see more clearly what they needed to do next. The song is as much a surprise for the character as it is for the audience watching their journey.

From the 'earning the right to sing' moment, comes pure unadulterated joy. It's a gorgeous surprise. It may not be the type of surprise that brings happiness and joy. Still, it's one that helps us to grow and experience vulnerability. It's a rare opportunity to experience our humanness and, for the first time, see life differently.

The modern concept of controlling everything that happens to us in our life prevents our ability to earn the right to sing. It means we dictate *if* we sing, *when* we sing, and *how* we sing. Goodbye to our sense of surprise, mystery and growth.

As humans, we're always riding on the wave. Our Peeps sit atop this undulating wave, and our breath brings this wave to life. The ebb and flow of life, of humanness, allows us to rest in troughs and strive in the peaks. The absolute climax of that wave trough and peak is our time to sing. Up there and down there, we've earned our right to sing. If we're always striving for and trying to control every part of our lives, then we're singing *all* the time. None of the songs are special anymore.

From my observation in the clinic with the women I treat, and from my personal experience, I believe all the adrenaline and cortisol we produce from trying to control everything, is killing us. I've watched as women become buried in the *'I must have it all,' 'I must be it all,' 'I must control it all,'* mindset, and end up with stress-induced illness and disease.

I am a recovering control addict. I almost died in 2019. Years of attempting to control every part of my life and dictating when I earned the right to sing made me depressed, anxious, and mere moments away from death. In my life, I'd completely lost my ability to breathe and experience the space that breathing allows us. And then an asthma attack almost killed me. My asthma attack was my *inciting incident*. Now I'd earned my right to sing. It got to the point of no return. In a life or death situation, it can go only one way or the other. You either go backward, which may mean death, or you learn your lesson from singing your song. You go forward in your humanness and the journey of your beautiful life.

What have been the inciting incidents in your life? Think about them. Write about all the awesome lessons you've learned about yourself from them.

I'm an A+type personality. I love the ocean or any body of water. Its movement, both subtle and gentle or loud and violent, brings me so much peace and joy. At my rock bottom, there was no movement left in my body. I made my body of water into a giant block of ice. Hard, stagnant, and unwavering.

**TRY THIS**

**When feeling overwhelmed by the stress of striving all the time, and trying to control everything, I do the following:**

**1.** Stop whatever I'm doing.

**2.** Place my left hand on my stomach. If I can, I place my right hand on my heart, too.

**3.** Relax the muscles in my face and breathe in and out.

**4.** Say hi to my Peeps. For some reason, when it's been a little while since I've checked in with my Peeps, I feel a little guilty and shy, so I'll be a little cute and funny. I greet them with a "Hey, how you doin'?" All 'Joey from Friends' style.

**5.** Listen to my Peeps, especially the ones in the background.

**6.** Tap about what my Peeps tell me.

**7.** Breathe in, "I love myself." Breathe out, "Yes."

**8.** I think about one little thing I can do now. It might be going to the toilet. It might be considering something concerning me. Or it might be to drink a large glass of water and find how it is cleansing my body and mind. It might be to sit still and continue my three anchors: Peeps, Tapping and Mantra until I feel calmer.

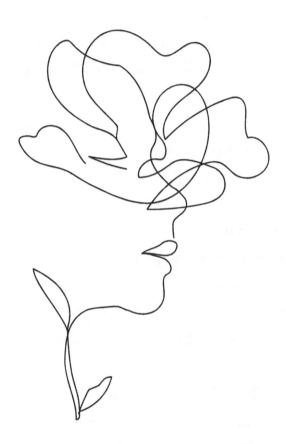

# Chapter Six

# I'M NOT SAYING DON'T GET ANYTHING DONE.

**I**'m not saying you're not allowed to have anything done at all. Given that I have performed over 18,000 treatments, that would be hypocritical. It would also be a sure-fire way to destroy my career while excluding the excellent methods you have at your fingertips to enhance your appearance.

As I've mentioned, none of the treatments I've performed over my career started with the patient wanting to begin their journey into cosmetic injections with the plan of becoming overfilled and over-frozen. On the contrary, they all started their journey saying things like: '*I don't want too much.*' '*I don't want it to be too noticeable.*' '*I don't want to look like the women I see on TV who look strange.*'

It's essential to work out why you want Botox and dermal fillers done and if they are for the right reasons or the wrong. My aim throughout this book is to teach you (just like I do every one of my patients) how to deeply know your beauty with or without the aid of cosmetic injectables. In a world that can be a little too gung-ho to overfill and over-freeze, what I'm asking you to do is consider *why* you want to have cosmetic injections done first and then every single time after that. It'll ensure you have realistic expectations of what cosmetic injections can do for you. It'll also help you recognise your very own Unique Facial Feature and nurture your Beautiful Unique Face. You need to know this because many practitioners out there won't know how to identify yours, let alone enhance it. Finally, you need to know how to determine if you're trying to heal something internal by getting stuff injected into your face. If you're trying to fix something deep inside by getting more stuff injected into your face, it's a recipe for disaster. It's a sure-fire way to end up with, not only an addiction, but also a face you don't like and which causes you heartache.

## When it's a good idea to have cosmetic injectables.

After you've read this book, I have the utmost faith you'll be in a position of empowerment and will make the right decisions about when to have your cosmetic injectables. **1. You will know what your Unique Facial Feature is. 2. You will have discovered and met your Peeps and have ongoing discussions with them. 3. You will know how to tap it out and ground yourself. 4. You will regularly practice your Mantra: "I love myself" (in breath) "Yes" (out breath).** You have your steadfast and stable Unique Facial Feature lighthouse guiding your way and your three anchors (Peeps, Tapping, and Mantra) adapting to support your ever-growing life. You have most definitely got this.

## CASE STUDY: KYLIE

Kylie was fifty-five years old when she came to see me after a recommendation from a friend and a family member. Her appointment notes read 'Very nervous.'

*I escorted Kylie into my treatment room. She studied me and my face thoroughly. Some patients do this. They want to examine my face intricately. I know why they do it. I let them do it. I welcome it. They're checking to see I'm not one of the overfilled and over-frozen faces. My face is, after all, an advertisement for my practice. If I look like one of the faces they see on TV or their Instagram feed that scare them, there's no hope for them to leave my clinic looking classy and natural.*

*"You look normal! That's such a relief," said Kylie.*

*"Yes, I do. It is possible to look normal."*

*"Good. I hate the way some women look when they've had too much."*

*"Yes, it's sad, isn't it?" I agreed.*

*"I've started to hate my face," Kylie said.*

*"Tell me why," I asked.*

Kylie told me she believed her wrinkles were out of control and she looked angry when she wasn't. She was feeling 'saggy' all over, but especially in her lower face. But her main reason for seeing me today was that she thought the wrinkles around her eyes were intense and, in her own words, she said her eyes were 'ugly.'

As Kylie spoke about her unhappiness with each of her facial features, I couldn't help, but be drawn to her eyes. They were what I'd describe as incredibly handsome eyes, in fact, almost sexy eyes. I think after you've examined thousands of faces in intense detail as I have, it's practically impossible not to find a person's Unique Facial Feature. Sometimes it's like finding the hidden treasure. When Kylie smiled, her eyes smiled too. You know the type. Eyes that smile and instantly make you want to smile too. Think Elizabeth Taylor, Gwyneth Paltrow, Meghan Markle and the natural version of Meg Ryan.

*"Your Unique Facial Feature is your eyes, Kylie."*

*"What do you mean? I have all these lines everywhere." Kylie said, pointing to the crow's feet around her eyes.*

*"Ah, but the little lines you have act as pretty little starbursts drawing all the positive attention to your eyes. If we take them away, your eyes will lose their attractiveness."*

*Kylie thought about this for a moment. "I had my crow's feet treated with Botox once."*

*"And what happened?"*

*"I didn't like it."*

*"Why?"*

*"I looked different."*

*"Exactly!!"*

We've already witnessed it with Stella. People with smiling eyes like Kylie and Stella always look different, and somehow worse, when they have their crow's feet treated.

*"I've always been such a happy person, but lately I don't feel it. People often ask if I'm angry or upset."*

What we needed to do was respect Kylie's smiling eyes. They were, after all, her lead actor. By fading out the features that were detracting from them, we'd make her eyes stand out even more.

*"Kylie, in all of us, our frown lines depict anger. Our forehead lines depict worry. The area of our lower face where the muscle is pulling down from the corners of the mouth creates a mouth frown. All of these are completely normal. But they all depict negative emotions, and for you especially, that isn't your personality. It's*

*why you feel like your face is betraying you as you get older. It's not showing the world, or you, who you are."*

*"Yes, I look angry and sad. That's how people treat me, so then I feel angry and sad."*

*"We need to focus on your Unique Facial Feature—your eyes. They're your lead actor. Let's examine which areas of your face are trying to pull focus away from your eyes. For you, it's the parts of your face that are making you look sad and angry; the opposite emotion your eyes depict when you are smiling. If we treat those areas, we make them fade into the background. Then they can get back to their job of supporting your lead actor. We want your eyes to shine and sparkle, just as nature intended."*

*Kylie looked in the mirror as I explained this to her.*

*"I had no idea that I had a Unique Facial Feature, let alone that it was my eyes. But it makes perfect sense. I've always been a happy and loving person, but over the last ten years, I feel like I've become sad and angry. Every time I look in the mirror, I see a sad, angry woman."*

*"Sadly, not many women know about their Unique Facial Feature."*

## *"I've treated myself so badly over the last ten years."*

*"I've made some awful choices over the last ten years because I've been so confused and upset about how I look. My diet is poor. I don't exercise. I don't do any of the things I used to love to do. I just couldn't work out why I looked so different."*

Educating my patients is the most important thing I do during our appointment together. If I can't teach them something that means they walk away feeling empowered and in control of their life, I feel like I've failed at my number one calling.

*"Now you know, Kylie, you have the reason why your face has changed, and you're looking sad and angry. You can feed your body the things it needs to make it your best body. You can care for yourself as you would care for someone you deeply loved."*

*Kylie began to cry.*

The emotional release of rediscovering you are beautiful and powerful is confronting. We often initially experience guilt from treating ourselves poorly, followed by a sense of delight once we realise, we have the power to change our lives from that day on.

*"This has been the best thing anyone has ever taught me. I feel like I'm in control now. I can make better decisions and be kinder to myself and feed my soul the things it needs to feel my best."*

I treated Kylie's frown, forehead, and lower face muscles with Botox. I placed a minimal amount of dermal filler in her mid and lower face. When Kylie returned two weeks later, she and I were thrilled. Again, I was struck by how handsome her eyes were, but even more so as her supporting actors returned to their place and allowed her eyes to take centre stage.

I adore what I do for work.

## *"I'm starting to have tickets on myself."*

*"Your eyes are beautiful, Kylie."*

*"I know! I didn't realise. But so many people have told me that over the last week. I'm starting to have tickets on myself."* *Kylie laughed genuine happiness.*

*Now that's what I like to hear!*

I have been treating Kylie for four years now, and her eyes still blow me away every time I see her. We have stayed true to her Unique Facial Feature, and Kylie is growing more beautiful each

174

year. She is feeling happy. There are times when Kylie compares her face to her younger self or gets sucked into believing she isn't enough, but she's empowered. She reminds herself that her eyes are unique to her, that she's beautiful and more than enough.

Kylie has discussed the concept of her Unique Facial Feature with her daughters and her friends. In doing so, she's encouraged them not to get sucked into the rabbit hole of comparison that leads women to have the same treatment as everyone else.

Staying brave on your journey, dear reader, is essential. Stay faithful to your lighthouse and three anchors. I'm proud of every brave woman who's had self-love and brought themselves back from episodes of self-loathing. We are in this together. Collectively we can ensure our lighthouse shines bright for us always. When we're lost, we only need to look for it, and there it is—leading the way. There will be times of immense temptation, as there are in all aspects of our life. But with the knowledge from this book, you can see the temptation for precisely what it is, a fleeting desire.

## When to avoid getting cosmetic injectables:

Look at the following statements, and if you answer yes to *any* of them, then you're having cosmetic injections done for ALL the WRONG reasons. Do the work in this book, then retake the quiz.

**1.** My friend/s have it done, and they tell me I need (insert cosmetic treatment) too.

**2.** The influencers I follow on Instagram look so happy after having their lips, cheeks, frown, forehead, and so on injected, I want to be happy like them too.

**3.** I think it will make me happy.

**4.** My partner told me I need to have it done.

**5.** I feel like I am missing out if I don't have it done.

**6.** There is a clinic doing fillers/Botox cheap, and I don't want to miss out on the deal.

**7.** A 'Botox party' sounds like fun! I could invite my friends, drink wine, and get a treatment discounted or even for free if my friends have enough stuff injected into their faces.

Interestingly, none of the above reasons sound too barbaric, do they? A few of them could be considered perfectly reasonable. In response to each answer above, here are the reasons why these are wrong reasons to ever have a cosmetic injectable treatment.

Let's examine each of these reasons individually:

## 1. *My friend/s have it done, and they tell me I need (insert cosmetic treatment) too.*

Response - your friends are not aesthetic medicine professionals and may only want you to have a treatment for two reasons. They've had their lips done and want you to share the experience with them. Or they have had their lips done and now think they are experts. Neither of which considers your best interest. It's the reason it's often a terrible idea to bring the all-encouraging persuasive friend with you during your treatment, and why 'referral to a friend' deals are unlawful. It's forbidden to entice people to have cosmetic injections done with the lure of you and a friend getting a discount.

Patient confidentiality can't be maintained as clinics will often ask their patients to refer a friend by providing the friend's name and email address, which is an unsolicited gain of information. The clinic then calls the friend (again unsolicited). And like announcing they have won something; tells them they have been referred by Janet Jones (breach of confidentiality) and can get their lips filled for 50% off. (Enticing to have a medical treatment with the promise of a discount.) There are so many illegal components of this commonly used system; I'm breaking out in a sweat writing this. One thing that annoys me more than women being turned into Pretty Ugly Faces is the people who ignore the rules put in place by our profession's governing bodies to protect the patient!

## 2. The influencers I follow on Instagram look so happy after having their lips, cheeks, frown, forehead, and so on injected, I want to be happy like them too.

Response - The influencers you follow on Instagram are often PAID to look 'so happy' after having their lips, cheeks, forehead and so on injected. They are always given the product for free in exchange for promoting the medical treatment and the clinic. If you were 'given' something worth $600 for free every few months, you'd be pretty chuffed, too! It's crucial to see Instagram and social media channels for precisely what they are; advertising forums. Places to sell an idea or a product. The modern-day sales rep is the influencer. Rather than going to the shops where we expect and accept that we'll be subjected to sales talk, in the guise of sharing, we're sold to in our own homes, our own private space, and during our personal time via social media.

So much FOMO comes from seeing posts by friends and influencers about what treatments they've had done. It can make us feel like we're not only missing out, but that we'll never know the secret to look beautiful if we don't get the treatment done as well.

Excellent and beautiful things happen on social media, too. Find more of that. The sharing of information to empower is brilliant. But if someone's sharing has made you feel icky, FOMO, and self-loathing, that deserves an unfollow in my book.

## 3. I think it will make me happy.

Response - The concern with looking outside of ourselves for something to make us happy is a very modern phenomenon. Sadly, nothing we do to ourselves, buy for ourselves, or are given will ever truly make us happy. It might briefly even make us feel worthy, but it'll be short-lived.

If we're unhappy, we need to find out why that is. You already know what I am going to say here. While talking to mental health professionals is incredibly important, that can often feel too far away for you or not something you need. The ones who can help you in an instant when you're feeling unhappy are inside you - your Peeps. If you look at a picture of some freshly injected lips, cheeks, jaw, chin and get a flash of inspiration thinking, "I'll get it done so it'll make me happy", STOP and lean into your Inner Power Practice.

With your Unique Facial Feature steadfast at the core, check in with your Peeps, ask why you are unhappy, and listen deeply to what they tell you. Tap it out. See what else comes up. Tap it out some more and then say your Mantra. "I love myself," "Yes." Work out from this what is making you unhappy and start planning what you can do to change that thing, so it no longer has that hold over you.

If we expect cosmetic injections to make us happy, we're not only setting ourselves up for guaranteed failure, but sticking a Band-Aid over a knife wound. Often if the treatment doesn't meet our expectations and make us happy, we'll blame our clinician.

We need to take responsibility for this. It's in our power to be realistic about why we're having treatment done. We can't expect to throw a rug over a floor that's collapsed with the hope it'll miraculously fix the floor. It'll look pretty for a while, and we can admire it from a distance. But don't, whatever you do, look too closely, let alone walk too close. You'll fall straight through.

## 4. My partner told me I need to have it done.

Response - This is a hard one for me to answer. So hard, in fact, I left it almost until the end of writing my book to complete. I can hear my father's words ringing in my ears. "If he/she told you to jump off the Story Bridge, would you?" You've read about my patient, Nessie, whose partner asked her why she didn't look like the women on his Instagram page. It led poor Nessie into a spiral of self-starvation that landed her a nice stay in hospital after her kidneys shut down.

Do men really have no idea the women posting their pics on Instagram are using insane filters that make them look NOTHING like they do in real life? Or is it that men are as confused as we are about what a real woman looks like?

Here I am going to go off on one, so I apologise in advance. Why are labiaplasties even a thing?! A labiaplasty is the cutting away of the inner labia so they don't protrude out of the outer labia. A few years ago, it was decided the appearance of these inner labia needed censoring in adult movies. So, to disguise the appearance of a normal woman's inner labia, a small censor square or two was placed over it. Voila, the labia are gone, and the outer vagina (bits you can see) appears all smooth and flush, no protruding bits ANYWHERE. Completely unrealistic and ever so dangerous. Next thing we know, men are wondering why their women don't look like this. Um, it's a censor square Einstein. Give me a censor square, and I'll happily place it over your mouth. Sorry, I told you this was a topic that makes me furious! When women who have no medical reason for the procedure but feel immense self-loathing for their bodies and girls as young as sixteen are heading to plastic surgeons requesting a 'designer vagina', I have a big problem.

Men are such visual creatures that some will often believe all they see. Women then start thinking there is something wrong with them. Feeling unworthy and self-loathing seems to be a typical headspace for women to find themselves in.

The first doctor to perform the labiaplasty was a disgusting man from Ohio called James Burt. **https://abcnews.go.com/ Health/ohio-woman-writes-book-love-doctor-mutilated-sex/ story?id=17897317 11/6/2020.** A gynaecologist with no surgical qualifications, from 1966, Dr Burt operated on women who genuinely needed post-childbirth procedures. While these women were under the effects of a general anaesthetic, and without giving consent, his colleagues turned a blind eye and Dr Burt would test out his techniques for rejuvenating their vaginal area.

He would perform clitoral circumcision and vagina reshaping in what he termed 'Surgery of Love.' This man decided that a woman's vagina was "structurally inadequate for intercourse" and took the liberty with her anatomy based on his warped views.

At this point in writing, I've practically ground my teeth down to my gums from anger at this man and his cronies. I need to step away for a bit and lean into my Inner Power Practice. James Burt died in 2012 after living to a healthy age of ninety-one. Hopefully, he is receiving his dues wherever his soul now rests.

So, if your partner tells you that you need to have cosmetic injectables or anything done, it's from a place of comparison rather than love for you. You must do two things. Firstly, lean into your Inner Power Practice so you know how loved and beautiful you already are, and secondly, please bid him farewell.

### 5. I feel like I'm missing out if I don't have it done.

Response - This is a common reason for having injectables done. To some extent, having a trusted friend recommend a practitioner is also a great reason to see the practitioner. Especially so, if your friend looks normal and you approve of the effects the treatment has made to her face. However, if you feel pressured into having it done based solely on the fact that you're missing out if you don't, it's the worst reason to have injectables done.

I have discussed FOMO in depth in Chapter Five, but the instant you feel you're missing out, there is only one thing you must do. Lean into your Inner Power Practice and think about what you think you're missing out on.

Is it the feeling of exclusion that is concerning you most? That you'll be the only one who isn't having it done and therefore, will no longer be accepted by your peers and friends? Is it that you're missing out on a secret that could make you more beautiful and, therefore, happy? Is it that if you don't do it now with your friends, they'll move forward quickly without you? Or is it that standing next to your friends you'll look ugly while they look beautiful?

These are all excellent reasons that your Peeps have revealed for your FOMO. They also provide a brilliant script for *Tapping it out.*

*"Even though I will have no friends left if I don't have my lips filled up, I deeply and completely love and accept myself."*

*"Even though I will be ugly if I don't have my lips filled up, I deeply and completely love and accept myself."*

*"Even though everyone will laugh at me for being a prude, I deeply and completely love and accept myself."*

*"Even though everyone will think I'm boring, stupid, judgemental and ugly, I deeply and completely love and accept myself."*

## 6. There is a clinic doing fillers/Botox cheaply, and I don't want to miss out on the deal.

Response - Why are they doing them cheaply? Ask yourself that first. I was at a cafe recently, and I couldn't decide between the freshly homemade vanilla slice or the freshly homemade caramel slice. The assistant told me they had another slice on special. It was double the size of the ones I was considering. And it was $5.00 instead of $5.95.

"Yes, I'll take it!" I said. Thrilled with my bargain, when it arrived, and I saw the wilted edges, hardened caramel on top, and dried out pastry base, I wanted to cry. A special treat for the family became not only a waste of $5.00, but was a disappointment for all, solely because I got sucked into a deal.

It's illegal to advertise package deals on social media to entice a patient to have a treatment they don't need. If a clinic advertises 3mls of dermal filler for the price of 2mls, or two anti-wrinkle areas for the price of one, the advertising guidelines committee at Instagram has deemed this is an unethical method of elicit advertising. Meaning, it is attempting to lure a patient who might not medically need the treatment to have it done purely based on them receiving the deal.

In Australia, it's illegal to advertise the pricing of scheduled medicines to the general public or your followers on social media. It turns the treatments with these medicines into a bidding war between clinics, which is not only unethical, but against the moral of providing medicine only to people who require it.

Oh yes, it's a hard area to navigate for the clinic, and the patient, isn't it? Because of the field of cosmetic medicine, in modern times, following more of a business model rather than a medical model, ethics can be easily blurred. After all, business

183

is all about selling as much of something to as many people as possible. Medicine is about following the problem-solving process and offering medical intervention, *only* to those who fit a strict criterion that clearly shows that they need it for their continued health.

If a clinic can provide amazing discounts, given we all acquire the medicines for approximately the same cost, they probably have the business model of getting as many bums on seats as possible. It ensures their cost of product, staff, and overheads are covered, but it reduces the time and care taken with each patient. You'll read more about this model in action in Chapter Eight when I introduce you to Amy.

Although the lines are easily blurred, it's not difficult to get it right. Consider, if a clinic is so comfortable to flout the law relating to medicines, where else would they be happy to cut corners? Your face, your aftercare, their emergency protocols? So yes, my stance on going to a clinic because they offer Botox and/or dermal fillers for a bargain is that you most definitely want to walk away from there in a hurry.

### 7. A 'Botox party' sounds like fun! I could invite my friends, drink wine, and get a treatment discounted (or even for free) if my friends have enough stuff injected into their faces.

Response - I love parties with my friends, I do. I especially love intimate gatherings at someone's house where bubbles are flowing, lots of fun conversation, plenty of giggles, and tasty nibbles to be had. However, this is not the environment needles, syringes, blood, body fluids, highly controlled schedule 4 medicines, and a myriad of potentially life-threatening procedures should take place.

Again, and back on my soapbox, Botox Parties are illegal. They'd be thrown out of court immediately for being shonky. Not only the practitioner and the company they work for, but the host too may also be responsible for any wrongdoing and complications, not if but when they arise.

Illegal fact #1 - No one can make an unbiased decision and give informed consent to have a treatment done when others are in the same room, urging them to have it, and more, done. There is a reason pyramid sales schemes use women to target women. Our friends easily influence us. Pyramid sales schemes have proven we're more easily influenced by friends and champagne than professionals who've done years of study in the field of skin.

Illegal fact #2 - Often, the host of the Botox party will receive a heavily discounted or free treatment, once the guests purchase a certain amount of Botox and dermal fillers. So, the incentive to make the guests have more and more medication, mostly that they don't need, is that the host gets a free set of lips.

Illegal fact #3 – There's alcohol present at these events. That immediately wipes out the ability to give and accept informed consent for a medical procedure.

Illegal fact #4 - For any medical procedure to be legally carried out, the strictest sterilisation practices must be upheld. All the surfaces must be cleaned to hospital standards. Current emergency drugs, including adrenaline and oxygen (via an oxygen cylinder) must be ready and available to be administered, if needed. All emergency policies must be available and prepared to be followed by all those present. On the small issue of oxygen, it shouldn't be transported within an enclosed vehicle. Meaning the practitioner must arrive at the Botox party with the oxygen cylinder tied securely upright, onto the back of a Ute, which displays a special permit stating that they are a licensed oxygen transportation service. Yes, I don't think many do this. I've never heard of any.

Consider your decisions before you make them. Sit with them. Spend time with them. Never fear taking time to respond. Sit back in curiosity and ponder a situation before deciding what to do.

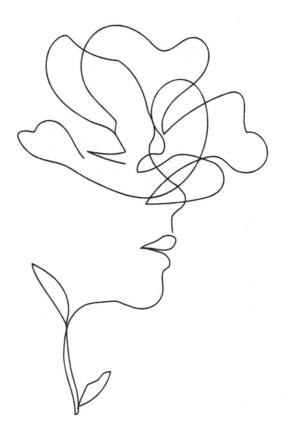

# Chapter Seven

# PRINCESSES AND QUEENS.

CASE STUDY: JOSEPHINE

Josephine was an acclaimed TV news reporter and journalist. Her journalistic talent identified in her early 20s, she'd been working for the same network for twenty years. Josephine started as a roaming news reporter, but quickly advanced to become the network's primary female newsreader. Night after night, she sat beside her male news-reading partner Mark and delivered the news to the nation.

The day after Josephine turned forty-five, the network's board called a meeting and discussed if Josephine would like to step into a more managerial role. Mentoring younger newsreaders and sourcing talent for the network. The new role included a surprising pay rise, more family-friendly working arrangements, and even the opportunity to work from home. It was an unexpected job offer. It left Josephine speechless, but suspicious. She thanked the board for the offer and promised to give them an answer within seventy-two hours.

## People felt it was appropriate to comment on her appearance.

Josephine had received trolling comments on her professional Instagram page and Twitter accounts. People felt it was appropriate to comment on her appearance, and some thought it was high time she stepped aside for a younger woman. One person even said they couldn't possibly believe the news with it read by someone who looked like her.

Josephine had her stable crew of supporters around her. Being a journalist, she was impartial to most things. Stoic, Josephine could let most things wash off her back.

Though over the last couple of years, Josephine believed her natural good looks were fading. She noticed her upper eyelids hanging lower than they used to. The network makeup artist needed to change the way she made up Josephine's eyes for the camera. Small jowls were forming in the once pristine line of her jaw. And, regardless of how well she'd slept, permanent indentations sat beneath her eyes, creating dark shadows and wrinkling skin.

After she left the network board meeting and surprise job offer and looked in the mirror, Josephine felt these changes in her face were even more prominent.

The meeting confused Josephine. She wasn't expecting a 'promotion' into a completely different role. Mark, her news-reading partner who was fifty, never mentioned he'd received a similar offer at forty-five. She wondered if perhaps he was considering leaving news reading, though she couldn't imagine it. She also couldn't believe that he'd consider it without discussing it with her.

Mark and Josephine possessed great onscreen chemistry ever

since their first screen test together twenty years ago. He'd told her everything important that was happening in his life. They were great buddies. Their families holidayed and celebrated birthdays together.

Despite her investigative journalism background, Josephine remained unsettled on the evening of the board meeting. She decided to sit with it for the evening, but it stirred uneasily like curdled milk in her gut. She spoke to her husband who suggested she call Sarah, her best friend. Sarah was the producer of a prime evening news and current affairs talk show. Sarah had been long trying to recruit Josephine to join her team. Her advice to Josephine was to watch and wait, something was about to change in Josephine's life.

## A younger version of herself was replacing her.

That night Josephine tossed and turned. She barely slept a wink. She went into the network much earlier the next day to do some research into a story that broke overnight in America. She was surprised to see the 'filming in progress' light on as she walked past the newsroom studio. Josephine walked into her office and turned on the monitor linked to the studio. She saw Mark reading the news from last night, with a woman she didn't recognise, reading her parts. The woman was much younger than Josephine, and the moment she formed this thought, Josephine felt like she might be sick. It sucked all the wind out of her and with that she realised, a younger version of herself was replacing her.

Over the coming days, Josephine considered all of her options. She called her agent and together they discussed her options. The advice again was to watch and wait. That something was about to change in Josephine's life. She didn't tell anyone at the network that she saw the younger woman screen testing with Mark. Her behaviour at the network remained the same as always. She was hurt and angry but understood it was not the younger woman's fault, she was forging her way in her career and had every right to test for the job of her dreams.

Josephine learned the young woman, Harriet, was the exact age Josephine was when she first read for the position. In the three years since completing her journalism degree, Harriet had been a war correspondent for a rival network. She was good. She'd be a great news anchor. Josephine didn't feel malice towards her.

For all Harriet knew, Josephine might've resigned from her post. Josephine, instead, discussed her options further with her husband and Sarah. Josephine sunk to her lowest low when she posted a picture of her outside the network on her professional Instagram page and applied the 'glamour' filter to the photo. Instead of the mix of comments discussing what news and current affairs she'd reported on the previous evening, people mostly commented favourably on her looks.

One person stated, "You look amazing, did you finally get some sleep?" Another said, "Your makeup suits you this way." And another said, "You've lost weight, you look great."

There wasn't one negative comment about her appearance, which had become commonplace over the last few years. Josephine wondered how people thought it was ok to comment on her appearance when she wouldn't dream of doing that to them.

Josephine felt guilty for lying to her Instagram audience about how she looked in the post. She understood she was a public figure and people wanted her to look a certain way, but that wasn't reality. Josephine couldn't turn back the years. She couldn't look like she was twenty-five when she was forty-five. Josephine couldn't apply a filter to the camera filming her read the news every night. She couldn't install a filter on her audience's TV screens. And, most importantly, Josephine couldn't sleep knowing she was applying a filter to the photos she posted on her professional social media pages. Josephine couldn't do that to all the women who needed to be reassured that, regardless of their age and their looks, they were enough. This was not who Josephine was prepared to turn into. She called a meeting with the board of the network the following morning. Her decision was made. She felt good.

The next morning, ever punctual Josephine was purposefully ten minutes late. She was busy removing the photos of her family from her office walls. There was a definite sense of expectation in the room as she entered. She deliberately didn't sit.

"I want to thank you all for the amazing opportunity you have afforded me. I'm honoured you think so highly of me that you'd like to promote me and have me mentor budding news presenters and journalists."

The tension in the room relaxed as the board considered their false victory.

Josephine concluded, "But I've decided not to take the position."

Suddenly the tension ratcheted up. The air stood thick with worry. Josephine waited a moment and said, "Now if you'll excuse me, I have an awful lot of important phone calls to make."

## What makes a Queen? What makes a Princess?

I don't know if there are any hard and fast rules to determine the difference. Still, I know that, at about the age of twenty-eight, I shifted in a phoenix-type way from being a Princess to become a Queen.

Today, at forty-five, I certainly feel more like a Queen than a Princess. It's more of a subliminal crossing that one day, I realised I was more a Queen than I was a Princess. Some say you need to endure emotional hardship to transition, but it may be a more positive inciting incident that is the catalyst for your transition from Princess into Queen.

What I want more than anything to be learned from this chapter is how it's essential to have your time as a Princess and then relish in your time as a Queen. Be happy to pass the baton with class and style.

Sometimes we want to hang on desperately to our time as a Princess. Some of us may never have shone as Princesses and feel we need to catch up. Or that we're owed that time. I believe that, once the time is gone, we are doing ourselves an injustice by hanging on to it. We have a much more exciting time to be had as Queens.

## Our Princesses need us more than ever.

They're lost in a world that sells the lie that perfect features bring happiness. They're of a different generation and are being fed so much utter rot on social media and reality TV. That it's acceptable and expected to look overfilled and over-frozen. That it's okay to have no respect for other people in the world. That it's natural to treat each other terribly. And to act from a place of anger and jealously rather than kindness and love.

> Queens, I call on you all; we have the opportunity to lead our Princesses. To be regal, classy, beautiful, as well as strong and peaceful. Be a leader. Adopt a Princess, in fact, adopt a few Princesses, a tribe of them, and guide them.

## Queens.

Now is the time to relish in our Unique Facial Feature. Although we've gone over how to discover our Unique Facial Feature, here is a quick refresher of how to find yours.

I'd rather you didn't ask someone what your Unique Facial Feature is. Think about you in your early to mid-twenties and remember how people described and complimented you. Did they compliment you on your beautiful eyes, amazing eyelashes, stunning hair, incredible cheekbones, cute chin, lovely nose, quirky smile, or sweet lips?

Think about someone in particular who impacted your life, who made you feel special. Who complimented you on a feature of your face? What was that feature? What did or do they love about your face?

Remember, when we're feeling *lost in our looks*, it's hard to remember anything positive that's ever been said about our appearance. You can quickly spiral downward into self-hate when you think about your appearance. Cast your mind back to a younger you, and the first thing that comes to mind about your face that others complimented you on. This is your Unique Facial Feature.

## Stop competing with other women. It's not a battle.

As Queens, we can nurture the Princesses in our community, not compete with them. When we see youthful women, we need to reassure them they don't have to have all the 'stuff.' They are so much more beautiful when they have less. The 'stuff' doesn't define who they are, just as it doesn't define who you are.

Queens know it's better to have nothing and feel full rather than have everything and feel empty. The energy we get from our Inner Power Practice is far more powerful than the energy we'll ever gain from adding more to our wardrobe or our face.

Talking to our Peeps allows us to sit in stillness as we will enable them to reply to and empower us. The energy we feel when we tap it out helps us to face the fear or anxiety that makes us feel unworthy and unattractive. The surge of loving energy our whole body feels when we say our Mantra, "I love myself" as we breathe in and "Yes" as we breathe out.

These are the things that give freedom from the expectation that we have to be, we have to look, and we have to feel a certain way. It's the practice that will relieve us from the expectation of achievement that's all around and gets us down with each birthday.

I know you look at yourself in the mirror and you see a different person looking back at you. She's not as spritely. Her skin isn't dewy and plump. You might have lines and spots and marks on your face that weren't there last year. There might be folds of skin that are hanging down, making you look sad. There might be lines etched into your skin that make you look angry or worried. You might look more like your older family members. You might even feel that you look less feminine.

Queens, what's happening to our faces as we age is all completely normal. If we accept that our fellow Queens are experiencing it too, we can feel solidarity and safety in numbers. Knowledge is power and, from a place of learning, we have discovered what our Unique Facial Feature is.

I want you to understand why and how your face is changing as you continue on your journey and settle deeper into your role as a Queen.

As a Queen, the lines on our face will become etched a little more into our skin. They tell the stories of our life. They're not evil, and we shouldn't think of them as our enemy. They are our storylines.

Remember in Chapter One when we talked about why the facial movement is so crucial for connection to others and yourself? Connection enables you to feel and give love freely. Connection allows you to surrender to the beauty of life.

Completely erase your lines, your facial movement, and you'll obliterate vulnerability and the real reason you're even here on earth, which is to feel. Ride the waves up and down. Rest in the trough, grow in the peak. Your Unique Facial Feature is still the same and, for many Queens, if they surrender to it their true beauty expresses itself.

We have forty-three muscles in our face. They all have a distinct purpose: to sustain life by eating and drinking. To be fair (and at a push) these only require eleven of the forty-three muscles. So, what's the purpose of having forty-three muscles in our face? Yes, to show emotion and communicate with others. We've been created with forty-three muscles to help us connect with others. By eradicating these with too much (or poorly placed) Botox, we erase our ability to love and be loved.

## What is happening to me?

It happens overnight, doesn't it, Queens? One minute you are feeling confident in the way you look, the very next you've morphed into a little old lady. All the Queens I treat in my practice feel this way, too.

> *"It seemed to happen so quickly." "I think it was when I turned forty." "This is what having children does to you." "Every birthday, I look about five years older." "I feel ok about myself, and then I see my reflection, and it ruins my day." "It's affecting my relationship with my husband/partner/children/friends." "I feel so ugly." "I can't tell anyone how I feel. I'm so ashamed." "Am I being vain?" "I don't know if there is anything that can be done." "Am I too far gone? Is this the end for me?"*

I hear these comments and questions daily from women desperate to know what to do and how they can look the best they can. Hopeful of gaining some sense of control back in their lives.

The lines in our face are perpendicular to the action of the muscle. So, if a muscle is an elevator and works vertically, like your forehead, it creates horizontal lines in your skin. If the muscle is a depressor and works horizontally, like our frown, it creates vertical lines in our skin.

Think of it this way. The underlying layers of your face are bone, muscle, fat, and skin. As we age, each of these layers, including the bone, gets thinner. Without the plump skin to bounce back, the effects of our facial muscles, our lines, become more prominent.

Strangely, the muscles in our face don't weaken like the muscles of our body. While I don't want to delve too deeply into anatomy, it's essential to appreciate that, above the bony layer of our face, we have ligaments that help to hold on to specific parts of our face. As we age, these ligaments become a little less taut. Meaning the tissue being held up by these ligaments end up collapsing a little further down the face. Think of the jowls and the folds between our nose and mouth. They occur because the ligaments holding up the tissue of our cheeks become a little lax. And that cheek tissue falls forward and down slightly.

JOSEPHINE CONTINUED.

## The Rule of the Queen.

Josephine called her agent and told her to call the network to let them know she wouldn't be returning but from what she'd seen, she fully endorsed their choice of Harriet to replace her. Then she called Sarah and agreed to meet with her to discuss her possible role in her news and current affairs program. Sarah was delighted for she knew how important it was to have someone like Josephine representing the voice of strong women worldwide. The voice of a Queen.

Then Josephine called Harriet and congratulated her on the new role. Harriet revealed that Josephine was her inspiration.

She'd dreamt of being like Josephine when she was just a teenager. She told Josephine the network had set her contract to start the following week and, much to Harriet's excitement, Josephine would be directly mentoring her.

*"You don't need me to mentor you, Harriet. I've read your writing and watched you. You have all you need already to be the best news anchor-woman for the network,"* Josephine said.

*"You are so kind; it means so much to me that you think that,"* Harriet gushed.

*Finishing the call, Josephine added, "Harriet, I won't see you at the network as today was my last day, but can you promise me something?"*

*"Yes, of course. Anything at all."*

*"Please promise me that in twenty years when your looks have faded and you find yourself in my exact position, that you afford the young woman taking your place the same kindness that I have shown you."*

Harriet didn't understand, for she didn't see the old, washed-up woman Josephine referred to, or the network and trolls saw. She only saw her strong and admirable heroine and a true Queen.

## Princesses.

You've got it tough. I know you do. Growing up, I had Dolly magazine. That was it. One pretty tame magazine that I would buy with my meagre thirteen-year-old bakery earnings. Mostly pages of fashion, but some pretty interesting articles for teenage girls about life, boys, friends, school, parents, family, and the world.

Then, as I got older, there were Cleo magazine and the international Cosmopolitan. Both a little more risqué. Some pretty hard-hitting articles. Again, lots of fashion and tips about hair and makeup. More advice about boys and sex, always from trained experts, though. Dolly Doctor was a great way to find out if things that were happening to me were happening to other girls, too. Our exposure to idealistic beauty was limited to supermodels and superstars. Cindy Crawford, Christie Turlington, Linda Evangelista, and Claudia Schiffer. Madonna, Penelope Cruz, Sharon Stone, and Cameron Diaz. Yes, they were beautiful. Although we could aspire to look like them and perhaps wear our hair like them, they were so far ahead of us, we knew they were up there, and we were down here. I'm not belittling myself or my generation at all. Quite the opposite. We had realistic expectations of what we could achieve. I never once thought I could be a supermodel, but that was ok.

Princesses these days though have a much tougher job. You're mere moments away from celebrity status, with your very own YouTube channels, your sudden influencer status, and your endless supply of credit for essentials like lash extensions, breast implants, lip filler, and Gucci handbags. The expectation of you is enormous. The peer pressure to look a certain way, behave a certain way is monstrous.

I see Princesses who believe having their nails, lashes, Botox, and dermal fillers are more important than buying food and essential medicine for illness. Princesses, whose only criteria for a man is the size of his credit card limit. Those dating men they neither like nor can see a future with, but men who'll spend money on expensive cocktails and the maintenance they're accustomed to. Princesses who are proud to be labelled *high maintenance*.

I watched a reality TV show in Australia recently. The first time two people see each other is when the bride is walking down the aisle to get married. A bride admitted being a 'high maintenance Princess.' She proudly told the camera how much she spent on Botox, dermal fillers, hair, nail and lash extensions, and an endless list of luxury items she considered essential. She and many other brides in the show insisted these things were necessary, and they wanted a man who could support their lifestyle. It was a sneak peek into the colossal pressure our Princesses experience. With identical hair and lash extensions, filled up lips, surgically enhanced breasts and noses, frozen faces, and far from kind personalities, they all resembled one another. Nothing unique about any of them.

The grooms disrespected the brides, the brides disrespected the grooms, and they all disrespected themselves. It was a societal train wreck.

The more our Princesses are fed the lies that reinforce the idea they're not enough and not worthy, the more they'll strive to do all the external stuff to themselves in the race to make them 'beautiful.'

So, while I worry about our Princesses and their flailing grip on what matters in their life to the detriment of their mental health, I worry as much about our Princes. A relationship based on appearances and material items is never a healthy and loving one. I've had many a young Princess and Prince tell me it's impossible to find a nice partner these days.

Princess, nothing external you buy or put in yourselves will help you live up to your expectations. You need to exercise your Inner Power Practice. You know what your Unique Facial Feature is. Turn off the device. Remove yourself from the situation and remind yourself of what is most beautiful about you.

Talk to your Peeps. Check in with them. Talk to the quiet ones. Ask them how they are, what they are feeling. Sit quietly and listen.

Tap it out. Tap about what your Peeps told you. See what else comes up.

Say your Mantra. Breathe in - "I love myself." Breathe out – "Yes."

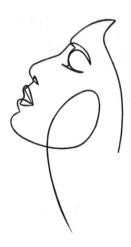

## Tips to be an honourable Princess.

**1.** Nurture loving relationships with family, friends, and partners.

**2.** Be with decent human beings. Remove yourself from those who aren't.

**3.** Treat others with kindness and respect.

**4.** Listen more.

**5.** Take the time to respond to things that make your heart flip-flop in both a good and bad way.

**6.** Sit with those things. Let the answers come.

**7.** Do not gossip. That icky feeling stays in your cells for days afterward. Gossiping is addictive.

**8.** Talk to trusted family members and friends.

**9.** Be a soundboard for trusted family members and friends.

**10.** Put someone who is kind and clever 1-2 steps ahead rather than someone loud and popular who shocks you with their behaviour.

**11.** Put yourself 1-2 steps ahead for a while. Watch your self-confidence skyrocket when you do this.

**12.** Know deep in your soul that this is your time. You are so special. You are incredibly loved.

With so much input coming at you 24/7, you are vulnerable darling Princess. Always remember, you are incredibly loved. I love you. All Queens love you, too.

Every Princess I see makes me melt with pure love. Every Prince I see makes me melt with love too. You are our future. I have the utmost faith in you to care for yourselves, us, and our world.

Princesses, find a Queen or two to adopt as your own. To be your mentor and provider of strength. Let a Queen nurture you while you relish in your special role as a delicious Princess.

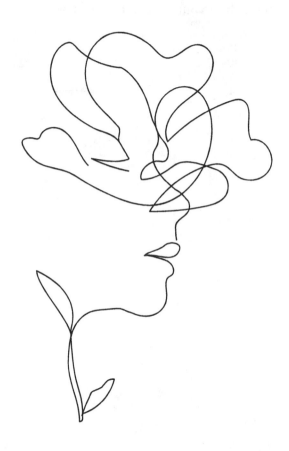

# Chapter Eight

## Part One

# SOCIAL MEDIA - LIKE BEING ON A FILM SET 24/7.

CASE STUDY: AMY

Twenty-two-year-old Amy couldn't believe her luck. On the train home from work, her phone beeped. Amy's friend had tagged her and a group of their friends in an Instagram post for a lip special in the Gold Coast.

The advert read:

*"End of Financial Year Special. Get the luscious lips that all of your Insta favourites have, without the price tag." "Only $395 instead of $550 for 1ml." "Tag 5 friends and if you all have treatment, you all get a free lip flip too." "Don't want the full 1ml? No problems, just bring a friend to your appointment and*

*split the syringe between you." "Only available for the next two weeks." "Get in quick, only available while stocks last."*

## Social media influencers with big lips all look so happy!

They secured their appointments via an Instagram message and were given the salon address. Amy and her friend took the following Friday off work and travelled the two hours to their appointment. Amy was so excited. Her lips weren't bad; in fact, they suited her face perfectly. Her face was sweetheart shaped, her eyes big and bright, her cheeks wide and pronounced, her mouth small with petite and nicely formed lips to match. Her face complete with a lovely pixie-like chin that acted like an exclamation mark drew your eye back up to her big, beautiful eyes. But as Amy scrolled through Instagram on her phone, which she frequently did, all she saw were luscious, big lips. All the influencers Amy followed who had lip fillers, were happy and loving life. Amy wanted to look like them and feel like them. Amy wanted bigger lips, too.

## The lip treatment was so quick.

In the salon, the gaggle of voices distracted Amy from the pain she felt when the needle went into her lips. It was a hair salon, and there were people everywhere, even lining up on the footpath to get in for the lip special. Although Amy and her friend booked their appointment for 1pm, they didn't have their treatment until 3pm. The treatment area was the staff lunchroom, so salon staff and various people came in and out while Amy had her lip fillers. It was someone's birthday. There was cake and the nurse laughed, sang happy birthday and was fed cake while she injected Amy's lips. Amy declined any birthday cake herself.

The woman doing the treatment introduced herself as a nurse. She'd told Amy the lip special was so popular she'd needed to order more product in. Her supplier sent it from overseas, and it arrived that very morning, hence the rush of people. Amy didn't ask what product the nurse was using. She didn't want to make a fuss. There were so many people, and Amy felt embarrassed when she winced the first time. She swallowed down the uneasy feeling she had. Fifteen minutes later, she was paying her $395 and walking past the line of girls gushing over her and her friend's new lips.

## I'm scared something has gone wrong.

Amy started to bruise on the drive home. Her friend didn't. Amy had a restless night. Her top lip and nose ached painfully. She was told she might be sore for the next day or two, so she took pain killers and tried to sleep. When Amy looked in the mirror the following morning, the skin between her top lip and the bottom of her nose was bruised. Amy messaged her friend. Her friend was just leaving the gym. She had no pain or bruising, and suggested Amy call the hair salon. Amy couldn't find a number to call, so she sent an Instagram message with a photo of her lips. Amy didn't receive a reply. The pain got steadily worse. She lay in bed with ice on her top lip and nose. She'd remembered the nurse had said to use ice to reduce swelling and bruising.

After Amy spent a few nerve-wracking hours googling her symptoms, she posted a message on the Instagram page of the hair salon where the special was first advertised. She asked if someone could get in touch with her as she was worried something was wrong. She didn't receive a reply. Later that day, Amy tracked down the salon's phone number from the neighbouring shop. She called them and was told the nurse wasn't there. She'd flown back home to Sydney last night, and they didn't have her number as it was organised through Instagram messages by a woman who knew their boss. They didn't know anything about Amy's treatment. Still, one of the hairdressers had bad bruising and pain too, and it settled a few days after her treatment. They were sure Amy's would, too.

## Social media is like being on a film set 24/7.

It's hard to imagine when I set out on my journey on that film set sixteen years ago, that I would be in this position today. My motivation to get into this industry all those years ago was to satisfy my confusion why a high-profile actress would change her appearance right before shooting the role of a lifetime. Little did I know back then, that within ten years, every single member of the general public would have access to the stuff that then, only celebrities and the uber wealthy could enjoy.

But now, we're a quick-fix society. It's not just quick; it's instantaneous. Instagram didn't exist on that film set, but now that it does, we're all as camera-aware and filter-savvy as Hollywood actresses of yore.

In a society struggling with meaningful connections because of the busyness of our lives, the resulting feelings of isolation and anxiety are often eased by the sense of belonging we get from social media. We rely on instant gratification to give us our hits of dopamine and pleasure. Often from meaningless and insignificant ways, such as social media and dare I say it, cosmetic injectables.

Excited from seeing the (fake) happiness we witness in others posting and gloating about their newly filled up lips, cheeks, and breasts, we anticipate the answer to happiness lies in those things (external fixers) for us. We willingly get sucked into getting our lips and cheeks filled or facial expressions frozen. It's a dangerous slope that leads to more obsession.

Like any addiction, healing requires some deep soul diving and time switched 'off' and away from the cameras. Some time away from scrolling through and zooming in on the parade of perfection on our handheld screens. It's like we're playing actor, director, and extra all at once: the power we have to make clips, photos, and be seen by the world are held in the shape of a phone. Once you had to make it in Hollywood for that kind of fame! But this access comes at a price.

Every day, minute and hour, we can compare ourselves to millions of glamorous strangers and picture-perfect influencers who, let me remind you, are paid huge amounts of money and endorsements to lie about how happy a product or service has made them.

## Social media forces you out of your now and shoves you into someone else's.

The other problem is that social media forces us out of the moment. We become trapped in someone else's portrayal of *their* now. Still, we know social media is not in any way, shape, or form a real indication of their life. It's an illusion, just like the movies once were. But the thing was, in the past, you could sit down to watch TV or go to the cinema and know you were about to experience an illusion. With social media, it's all masquerading as real life.

I see the 'happiest' social media influencers as private paying patients in my clinic all the time, and they are not like that in real life. They are wrought with anxiety, stress, panic, and fear of judgement. They are continually assessing how they will be perceived, like once only actors were. And they post for likes and attention rather than honestly sharing their lives. They are mini TV commercials, actors playing a role. It's causing all of this confusion and mental unrest because people think Instagram is real.

Actors wouldn't get a job in an audition for a skincare product which claimed to change your life if they said, "Don't be ridiculous. This skincare product can't fix your life." Fear sells and, in this day and age, the biggest fear is the fear of missing out.

I have a patient who works for a skincare company and uses my own formulated skincare products and *not the products she sells to the public.* Why? Because I based my skincare on research and medical therapeutic guidelines rather than hype, hearsay, luxurious packaging, a pyramid of social pressure, and an influencer being paid to say that it works. Am I comfortable with my patient doing this? No, not at all. It sits uncomfortably in my gut. This patient is mostly lying to her customers, but then again, she is expected to have great skin and sell the idea of great skin, which is impossible from using the products she sells. I am compliant in her betrayal of society.

Every day I'm approached by 'influencers' and influencer agents who tell me they've identified me as a high-profile business, and they can increase my customer base and business turnover. When this happens, I'm being asked to supply class-A drugs to the dealer who will stand outside the school and on sell to the school kids struggling with the confidence in their looks. They're asking me to exacerbate a society in crisis. To sell all this on the promise of an increase in money and earning potential is not only medically unsafe but unethical and immoral.

## Performance anxiety is no longer just for actors.

Many influencers I've treated as patients are on a multitude of anti-anxiety and antidepressant medications. They are Princesses who feel this particular Instagram-perfect look is the only way they can earn money.

Behind closed doors, the professional influencers suffer the damage of performance anxiety. Their mental and physical health suffers because they are continuously watched and judged. Scared to make a wrong move, it's impossible for them to relax. Bound to the idea that they must be perfect, they no longer know who they are or what they want. They're expected to be the face of perfection and promote all sorts of products and services, often from competing brands. It's a logistical and moral nightmare.

During my Masters of Acting thesis on performance anxiety (also called stage fright), I conducted a study on actors, singers, dancers, and professionals who were called upon to give oral presentations. I researched ways to overcome performance anxiety. I found that one of the most successful methods was visualisation. We are so adept at thinking ourselves into a way of feeling.

Sadly, we often use this storytelling ability to conjure up the worst possible scenarios in our heads. We then release cortisol which tells our brain, vital organs and muscles to get ready to run because there is an imminent threat and we must protect ourselves. And this is before we've even stepped on stage! We make ourselves ill purely from imagining ourselves doing something.

During my study, I watched incredibly talented performers and professionals, paralysed in the wings, unable to move or breathe let alone take their place on the stage for their scene or their speech. The physiological effects of performance anxiety are akin to someone having a heart attack. If you were to take the person out of their environment, and place them on the street, an ambulance would be en-route to assist them.

## Paralysed with fear.

We're now experiencing this level of performance anxiety in our homes, in our work, and in every facet of our day as social media infiltrates every crevice of our life. We're told we need to be smashing it, making a fortune, hustling, winning, and beating our competition into the ground. Making money while we sleep, becoming entrepreneurs, waking up earlier than everyone else, exercising daily, eating better, and thinking only positive thoughts. And we are told we need to control our thoughts, our actions, and how others perceive us.

The idea we are never good enough is continuously reinforced. The need to perform is with us always. We don't know where the stage starts and where it finishes. We're always on show. Never a time to stop and relax. Even the time we have dedicated to a holiday, a time to relax and switch off with loved ones, is on show and is being judged. Akin to Charlie Brooker's *Black Mirror*, every breath we take in life is being rated. We can never just *be*.

The constant need to compete, to look prettier (and it is a warped idea of pretty at best), and to attain perfection, is killing us. This is the effect that our current addiction to social media, and the feeling that we are not good enough, has on us. When we have more reasons to be content than ever before (mentally, physically, and socially) yet still struggle this way, we must realise we are in a time of crisis and chronic stress.

If only we could stop anticipating the worst for the future, regretting the past and beating ourselves up over things we have or haven't done; we might appreciate the air that fills our lungs and experience the absolute beauty in now.

---

Knowing and trusting in our lighthouse - our Unique Facial Feature - and spending some of our precious energy on our Inner Power Practice including our three anchors of Peeps, Tapping, and Mantra - will save us and bring us back to our beautiful now.

---

AMY CONTINUED.

## It hurt too much to cry.

Three days after her treatment, it was Monday, and Amy's top lip and nose were so painful and swollen she had to call in sick to work. It looked like the top layers of skin were peeling off. It hurt too much to cry, so Amy tried not to.

*Amy contacted my clinic and told my receptionist her story. My receptionist asked her to send some photos through to our mobile number, which Amy did. Ten minutes later, I called Amy and asked her to come in immediately. Within minutes of Amy arriving, I injected a high dose of product to dissolve all the dermal filler in her lips. Amy had a vascular occlusion which was leading to tissue necrosis. It needed to be fixed immediately, otherwise, Amy was at risk, not only of permanent scarring, but losing her top lip and her nose. Amy's throat tightened. She thought she might pass out.*

## "I nearly lost my nose."

*Within ten minutes, the pain in Amy's nose and lip lessened. The skin around her top lip and nose started to pinken, and the blueish tinge faded a little. I told Amy she was very, very lucky. Blood supply was now getting to where it had been blocked off. Amy and my clinic staff were delighted, but this was only the start. Amy stayed in my clinic for the next two hours. We checked on her regularly. She returned to me four hours later to have more dissolving treatment.*

I started Amy on antibiotics, and she returned to my clinic for the next two days for further dissolving treatments.

## *"I would never have treated your lips."*

Amy noticed that our lip fillers were $500. As she looked in the mirror at her face, she told me she wished she'd come to me in the first place for her lip fillers. I told Amy, given her eyes were her Unique Facial Feature I wouldn't have treated Amy's lips. Instead I would have further enhanced her beautiful eyes with a treatment that cost $100. And, at most, some of my medical skincare to reduce a couple of her acne scars. Amy was speechless.

I didn't charge Amy for any of the dissolving treatments or the care that I gave her over the three days. I was so happy that Amy had been brave enough to call us and ask for help. We both teared up when we compared the photos of Amy on Monday to her face after the dermal filler was gone, and her skin was less swollen, mottled, and blue. I was just relieved I could reverse Amy's necrosis.

After three days, Amy was well enough to return to work, but the skin had broken down into a crusty wound that covered her whole top lip, the skin above her lip, and the tip of her nose. Amy was too embarrassed to see her work colleagues and boss, so she called in sick for the whole week. Amy went to see her GP and cried throughout the appointment. She sent her Sick Certificate to her boss.

## Three months later.

Three months since Amy jumped on the 'end of financial year lip special' and she was still suffering the damage of her discount lip treatment. Amy had spent thousands of dollars on surgical treatments, laser, and creams to reduce the scarring. Her skin would never be where it was before she had the lip fillers. She was likely to have permanent scarring and residual pain forever.

Amy was getting through the emotional hurt of her ordeal. Still, her self-confidence was in tatters, and she started to see a psychologist once a fortnight.

Amy never tracked down the 'nurse' who did her lip filler treatment, and the hair salon where her procedure was performed, denied any responsibility. Amy had a lucky escape but the effects will be with her forever.

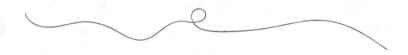

# Part Two

# THE JOY OF FAILURE

## CASE STUDY: ANITA

**I**'m someone who's always felt the need to make people like me to prove my worth. I believe it comes from my early childhood. In primary school, we moved a lot, at least once every 6-18 months. The longest I ever stayed in a school was eighteen months. Every time we moved, I needed to make new friends and 'pitch' myself to my teachers and peers to prove myself worthy of their love and attention. I was always starting from the beginning again and again, and I worked out that the best way to make people happy was to make things perfect for them.

After two boys, my father desperately wanted a baby girl, so, when I was born, everyone rejoiced. It was their perfect gift. Relatives quickly named me "Little Miss Perfect" and "She who could do no wrong." Little did they know the price that seeking out perfectionism would have on my life.

## I needed to make it better.

It wasn't until my chance witnessing of the director and makeup artist that I considered how injectables, which prevented actors from being able to show emotion on their faces, meant they couldn't tell a story and connect with their audience.

Botox was a relatively new phenomenon, and I needed to know more about it. I understood that women and men wanted to delay the visible effects of ageing by softening wrinkles and replacing lost volume. In 2004, actors were much more likely to seek age defying, face and body enhancing treatments than non-performers, and then female performers much more likely than their male counterparts.

The pressure on looking good is immense for female performers. Although I've been fortunate to have had performing jobs in theatre, film, and television, I've also received a truckload of rejections based entirely on my appearance.

As a performer, you're shortlisted for an initial audition based on a close-up and filter-free 8x10 inch photograph of your face, with reference to details of your physical size. On a performer's CV, listed right next to your name, are the measurement of your dress, bust, waist, hip, and height. Talk about pressure to conform to the idea of ideal beauty. Regardless of past performing experience, training, or skill, your appearance as a female performer is the most likely aspect to win or lose you a role.

## *"Your nose is too big."*

The level of scrutiny on an actor's appearance is intense. And it takes its toll. I was once rejected for an acting role because my face was "too thin." At the time I was 47kg and size 6, which was exactly what the same director wanted in my bodily appearance, so it wasn't like I could "fill out" only on my face and have it not change my body. If it were today, I could've had dermal fillers to fill out my face. I often wonder what I would've done if Botox and dermal fillers were as readily available then, as they are today.

## My NOSE obsession.

I understand the pressure. I always hated my nose. Felt it was way too big for my little face. I obsessed over it. I'd planned that the minute I was eighteen, I would take out a loan and have a nose job. If I were eighteen in today's society, I probably would've done the Afterpay option and had it done on my eighteenth birthday. I was depressed about my nose. When I was ten, my brother had Madonna posters plastered all over his bedroom wall. I remember being at a bus stop, going to school around this time, and planning my escape route away from my nose. "If I can just make it to eighteen, I can get surgery and have a nose just like Madonna." Changing my nose was my main incentive for becoming an adult.

When I reached eighteen, however, I had no money even to entertain the idea of getting a nose job. Then, once I finished university, I was determined to save to buy a house. No spare money here for a nose job, I'm afraid. My dissatisfaction with my nose was always front and centre of not only my face but of my mind, too. However, the thought of spending the deposit for a house on getting my nose made smaller, felt ludicrous to me. I saved my deposit and bought my house, but my nose obsession was always there to haunt me. I am so grateful that social media wasn't around when I was younger. I can only imagine I would have screenshots of the noses I pined for clogging up my phone's memory. Instead, I had cut-out magazine pictures.

Once I moved to the UK at twenty-three, although I still obsessed about my nose, the possibility of being able to afford a nose job was even less likely. Then, I scrubbed in on a surgery where a woman had a rhinoplasty, and it took the shine off considerably. While I hated my nose, I didn't hate it that much to put the poor thing under the physical trauma of a rhinoplasty. Over the next couple of years, I went on a merry-go-round of hate and acceptance of my nose.

I graduated from drama school and quickly realised my nose got me typecast into every role I secured. Never one to be cast as the beautiful lead, they always cast me as the professional woman, the expert, the lead actor's all-knowing, wise best friend. My nose seemed to portray the illusion my character was intelligent and wise. I was doing okay in terms of getting acting gigs, and my agent told me it was my nose, along with my acting ability (ahem) that cast me so well!

I once had a man tell me that my nose was gorgeous. I laughed at him. 'Gorgeous' is an adjective I would never have dreamed could ever be used in the same sentence as my nose. I assumed he was drunk.

My nose and I could do okay, but one thing would spiral me into a wave of hate for it. After three callbacks and successful auditions, they rejected me for a regular part in a TV series because the executive director felt my nose was "too big" for the role. I'd always been self-conscious about my nose, so losing out on a significant role because of it confirmed my fears.

I cried as I searched Google for plastic surgeons. I cried even more when I saw the average price of the surgery. I was a small-time performer who was struggling to meet the expectations of directors on my appearance. I could only imagine how big stars handled the pressure of expectations on their appearance. When you're employed based on your looks and an influential decision-maker tells you a physical part of you isn't good enough, it's hard to remind yourself that the one thing that they don't like, is the exact reason another director might cast you. In search of the perfect and most employable face, actresses seek to get each facial attribute 'fixed.'

When our favourite actresses and actors started using Botox and dermal fillers and plastic surgery, the whole world noticed. What followed was a barrage of commentary from society on whether we approved.

I hated my profile because of my nose, and if I sensed someone was looking at me from the side, I would always turn to face them. I learned this skill when I was a teenager and I carried it through to adulthood. On my first date with my now-husband, I wouldn't let him see me from the side. I think I even told him he wasn't allowed to look at me from the side on that first date. It was exhausting, turning my head always to look at his face to stop him from seeing my profile. Thankfully, after almost seventeen years together, I'm not so precious about my nose and even believe him when he tells me he loves my nose.

I still look at other women's noses and sometimes pine after a smaller, more delicate one to suit my face. With so many options available to us today, it's no surprise we believe the perfection of our facial features will improve our life.

## Confusing perfection with happiness. How perfection almost killed me.

At most cosmetic medicine conferences I attend, friends and colleagues, new acquaintances and strangers, feel the need to tell me I need work done on my face. My lips are "too small", my cheeks "too flat", my forehead "too lined", and my frown "too strong." It takes a lot of courage, but I thank them for their concern and comment that I am ok the way I am. All while looking at them wondering where they lost their barometer.

About five years ago, at a conference in Sydney, I noticed a dramatic change in the appearance and behaviour of the other attendees. Almost a frenzy of perfected features. When did they stop seeing what was normal in their face and start trying to chase all the lines and all the hollows the hell out of town? When did they become so obsessed with perfecting everything? I noticed at yearly conferences, regardless of how much they had pumped into their faces, it didn't make them happier.

Something was seriously amiss with this formula of perfecting all the facial features. I felt like an outsider. I found it difficult to connect to others at the conference. Was I being ostracised for having facial movement, displaying emotion and for having far-from-perfect facial features? Or was it just so hard to create a connection with them due to their frozen and overfilled faces, that I felt alone? The desire for perfection had hit fever pitch amongst the clinicians, which meant the storm was about to erupt for the patients of these clinicians.

It was easy for me to see what was happening to them and want the complete opposite for myself. I have a pretty realistic view of the industry and can step back from it and observe it from a healthy distance. It is, after all, the experience of seeing the lead actress in the enviable position of a juicy acting role that I could only dream of, jeopardise it all with a frozen and overfilled face that set me on my journey in 2004.

## Everyone looked normal.

I remember leaving that fever pitch conference five years ago, arriving at the airport with one of my closest allies in the industry, a dermatologist and physician, and we both exhaled in relief as we watched 'normal' people go about their business. Surrounding us were normal-looking people, normal expressions, and beautiful unique faces. Faces that moved in ways you expected them to move. We instantly felt a connection with the strangers around us.

We could see when someone was happy because their crow's feet crinkled in delight. We could tell when someone was sad or worried or even angry because their foreheads moved appropriately.

"These people are my people," I said to my friend. "Mine too," she replied. Wow! We were in a conundrum. Two successful practitioners of cosmetic medicine, pining for wrinkles, small lips, and flatter faces. We simply weren't willing to join the trend of following our clients down the rabbit hole of perceived perfection and Pretty Ugly Faces.

> As a perfectionist, my revelation on that day at the airport, was that I would perfect the art of making my patients look imperfect. For *that* is truly interesting and beautiful. It allows them to remain connected to others and themselves, experience vulnerability and love. None of my patients would leave my clinic with 100% perfected facial features.

## The Beginning Of The End.

In August 2019, as my illness manifested and on the eve of the day that changed my life, I lay in bed and scrolled through Instagram. A cosmetic clinic posted a picture of a woman of indiscriminate age pouting excessively. She could have been twenty or sixty years old. It was impossible to tell from her grossly unnatural and puffed up facial features. Her lips, cheeks, chin, jaw were all puffed up with excess dermal fillers. Her crow's feet, frown, and forehead lines non-existent. The caption on her photo said, "Today is the happiest I've ever been with my face," like commenting on a batch of cookies she'd just baked. Your face is something you should love forever, not have only a fleeting romance with on a sunny day in 2019 when your freshly injected lips are still swollen and bruised.

Her next photo was a 'before' photo of her face, only a year prior but barely recognisable as the same person. Her features were looking natural and, to the trained eye, only slightly enhanced. She was smiling in a social situation—genuine happiness in her uniquely beautiful eyes. As a clinician, I saw what I see in many women who believe freshly injected lips or cheeks or chin or whatever will make them happy, and that's deep sadness. I could see she was a deeply troubled young woman despite saying she was the happiest she'd ever been. She was under the illusion her newly inflated facial features would make her live up to the external expectation of what was considered beautiful. And she'd feel worthy of loving herself and being loved by others.

This belief wasn't isolated to this poor woman. I saw an alarming rate of my own and other's patients pursuing perfection like their lives and happiness depended on it. I felt responsible for setting them right. Making them understand these things don't come from within the syringe, but from within them. It was incredibly depressing. I fell asleep, but awoke from a horrific nightmare.

## Blood, pus, glitter, Botox and dermal filler sprayed everywhere.

*My eyes are stuck shut, and I'm soaked in sweat. Delirious, I spiral uncontrollably into a frightening rabbit hole. My heart races, my blood pressure skyrockets, a crushing ache in my chest, grips me, and then they start. THE FACES.*

*Faces come hurtling at me in the dark. Desperate faces beg me for more. Crying, hysterical, screaming, poking, pulling my hair, they pick bits of skin off me and flick them into my gasping mouth. They reach into my chest and squeeze my heart hard.*

*Their giant smiling mouths with blindingly bright white teeth protrude while bulbous eyes weep crocodile tears of sadness, their tarantula-like eyelashes slicing painfully through my eyeballs. Almost too pretty, grossly perfected features on distorted faces push hard into my own. Their swollen and oozing lips can no longer pronounce words. Sharp cheeks, pointy chins, razor-sharp jawlines, and tiny, almost non-existent noses make breathing impossible.*

*I become weak. I've no fight left. The faces are winning. They strangle me, sit on me, straddle my mouth and nose. Finally, their petrified faces blow up like pufferfish and explode—blood, pus, glitter, Botox and dermal filler spray everywhere.*

*"NO!" In a final attempt to escape the faces, I rise out of the rabbit hole. From this perspective, I can see them all.*

*Thousands upon thousands of Pretty Ugly Faces. The PUFs become angrier and more desperate as they realise I'm getting away.*

*I deny them, abandoning them, and they're both furious and heartbroken. I feel sorry for them and momentarily contemplate going back to help. Logic reigns.*

*I must escape. They scratch me with knife-sharpened fingernails that remain lodged in the flesh of my legs as I kick myself from them and float away.*

*Barely audible, I hear the PUFs scream in unison:*

*HELP!*

I woke suddenly from that dream, feeling unwell and unable to breathe properly. I felt the virus take hold in the forty-eight hours prior and knew it would go one way or another. I took some steroid medication to reduce the swelling and irritation in my airways, doubled my inhalers and painkillers. My husband looked at me, and I knew from his face that I was in big trouble.

"You look really unwell."

"I feel awful," I answered.

He touched me, "You're burning up."

"I can't breathe."

"You can't work like this."

"I have to work. I have to see my patients."

The understanding I was too unwell to work, and that I would need to let my patients down crashed into me, and I started to cry. Crying when your airway is already severely compromised with illness-induced asthma is not wise. Still, by the time my logical brain tried to override my emotions and rein them in, it was too late. I had a full-blown asthma attack—my first and hopefully my last.

Unable to breathe in or out, total silence replaced my crying. The sensation started leaving my fingertips, feet, and face. My mouth tingled, and my face felt cold. My husband and our bedroom went black. I collapsed on the bed, clutching my throat, unable to get any air in or out. "Nebuliser," I mouthed to my husband.

The next part is a bit of a blur. On the brink of unconsciousness, somehow, we got some Ventolin into my lungs. My husband assembled the nebuliser I'd bought four years earlier when I last had illness-induced asthma and got some hospital grade medication straight into my airways.

My husband started to call an ambulance, but I convinced him I wasn't dying. I showed him I could take little breaths in and out and that perhaps he might instead call our GP surgery and see if I could get an appointment sometime later that day. After I'd finished treating all my patients.

However, thirty minutes later, and in our GP's consulting room, our normally jovial family doctor sat in front of my husband and me. She was furious we hadn't called an ambulance and threatening to do so right then to have me admitted to ICU. My husband had just finished telling her I was worried about letting my patients down if I couldn't treat them today. My GP was exasperated and angry.

"You almost died this morning and all you're worried about is seeing your patients?! *They* will not die if you do not treat them today or tomorrow or ever, but *you* are dying. You are moments away from being intubated, and in a coma. You have almost no air entry into your lungs. I feel like putting you in the hospital just so that you understand how desperately ill you are."

It was then that my husband broke down and told our GP I wasn't coping with life. He was right, of course. I wasn't coping. I hadn't been coping for some time. My asthma attack was the last straw for my husband.

### *"I need to keep my patients safe."*

I returned to my GP on Monday to be told I wasn't allowed to go back to work that week. She didn't understand. I needed to get back to work. I needed to ensure women were not taken advantage of by their social media feeds and unscrupulous practitioners who continually fed them the lie that they were not beautiful enough without the lips, cheeks, chin, and so on.

I believed it was my responsibility to my patients and the women in society disheartened by the growing number of pretty ugly faces. The pressure I felt was immense. While the frenzy on social media was perfect facial features, my behaviour was just as frenzied. To believe I could save all the people from this lie was absurd.

My GP was angry with me.

"You are dying," she said. "You are so close to dying from the stress of trying to help everyone. You have to stop now, or you will die! We need to get your work-life balance sorted."

It struck me then; I have access to all the stuff that women are being led to believe will make them happy, and yet, I am this miserable. I have access to all the Botox and dermal fillers you can imagine. I mean, all of it! If I wanted to, I could have 5000ml of it injected into my face right now. But it won't make a spot of difference to how I'm feeling.

## My new diagnosis.

*'Anxiety, panic attacks, and reactive depression in the context of running her own professional business, mother to two girls, wife, etc.,'* was the diagnosis I walked away from my GP with that day.

Having my lips plumped wouldn't touch the surface of what

was eating me up because guess what? The more we try to bury it with changing the way we look, the more we avoid the internal work we need. The more the bastard comes up to the surface and bites us firmly on the nose. If I thought that buying the lips could make me happy, well, I'd have all the lips by now.

## *"Everyone is better off without me."*

I would lie awake at night, not for worrying about my husband or daughters, but worrying instead about how I could keep my patients happy. My obsession with this impossible task soon escalated to the belief I was a failure at every aspect of my life. I was a bad mother, wife, daughter, sister, and friend.

In hindsight, that frenzied conference I attended in Sydney five years earlier when I noticed it had hit fever pitch, was the start of it. If the clinicians performing the treatments were being sucked into the lie of perfected facial features, it would only be a matter of time until their patients and society at large caught on.

I was failing miserably to convince everyone that what they saw on social media was a lie. Then I realised I could no longer care for and make people feel better; it just wasn't working. My belief about myself was being tested. I seemed to fail at everything in my life. But mostly, I was failing me.

My husband was better off without me because he was a solo parent most of the time. He was the nurturer in the family because, as any business owner knows, I was always working, stressing. I was also trying to make it perfect for my patients. My husband witnessed my "everyone is better off without me" meltdowns, which is why he told our GP I wasn't coping with life.

I couldn't think of a way to get off the spinning wheel of trying to meet everyone's expectations. Rather than just admit I couldn't make it perfect for everyone, I thought about ending it all. Instead of accepting the love I was surrounded by, I couldn't forgive myself for the insane pressure I'd put myself under.

## The gift of my near-fatal asthma attack.

So, you see, while my near-fatal asthma attack was the closest to death I've ever been, it also brought me the closest to a life I've only dreamed about. My inciting incident challenged all my beliefs and made me steer a new course for my life.

## The joy of failure.

Failing is an incredibly powerful gift. The main thing that's changed in my practice and my life since my near-death experience, is that I ask patients to take control of their happiness. Their happiness is *not* my responsibility, nor the responsibility of the Botox or dermal filler; It's theirs.

We can all grow up, see social media for what it is, put our big girl pants on and accept our happiness is a journey, and we are at the helm. I teach my patients what their Unique Facial Feature is, and what makes their Beautiful Unique Face. It doesn't matter how much stuff they have injected; they won't be happy unless they do the internal work. I also discovered I needed to write my book to get my message out there to the masses because I was burnt out, I was done. In person, I am one little voice, but on paper, my voice is huge and can reach millions of women who need help.

## The foundation of my Inner Power Practice.

I have made an enormous discovery over the last year. My body and mind have failed me in a million and one ways. I have been more ill than I have ever been before in my life. I hadn't listened to my body when it desperately needed to stop and rest. I have carried unrealistic burdens upon my back and fallen in a heap beneath the weight of them.

I have made the stark realisation that I am far from perfect. I believed everything I did as a mother, wife, daughter, sister, and friend was wrong. My striving for perfection has meant I have become the most imperfect and vulnerable version of myself.

I have always been ashamed to show vulnerability and imperfection. My nickname was 'Little Miss Perfect.' How could I not live up to this expectation? This last year my perfection erupted, all messy, fearsome, destructive and hot. Just like a volcano, it still rumbles beneath the surface worryingly. Which means I do the internal work I teach you here in my book, thus reducing the risk of another explosion, or I hand out hard hats to all around me.

In April 2019, four months before my asthma attack, I took myself off to a conference in Monaco and then onto an 8-day women's retreat in Italy. It was an incredible experience. I knew no one there, but the call to travel to the other side of the world to be part of this retreat was so strong, I travelled the 16,000kms not knowing what was waiting for me. I danced, lay, cried, hiked, sang, drew, and wrote with twelve other women who'd come from every corner of the earth. Each of us felt similar callings to attend the retreat. Each of us possessed incredible and heartbreaking stories that led us there. I have never been as vulnerable as I was amongst the women with whom I shared the retreat. I was frightened, ashamed and so vulnerable. The main thing that continued to come up for me was the huge expectation of being perfect for everyone. Around the room, the women told me what they saw in me. It was so different from what I saw in myself. They saw someone who made them laugh. They saw someone who had deep thoughts and who was incredible. No one saw the failure I saw in myself or the inability to live up to my expectations of myself. They didn't see my uncontainable self-loathing.

Our days started at 7am and finished at 10pm. Meditation was a huge part of my retreat. On the fifth day of the retreat, Tues, 5th April 2019, we hiked to a spiritual site in Quarna Sopra. We stood in a circle, closed our eyes, and focused on our breathing. I would really love to tell you what we did then, but I'd be making it up because I have no idea what happened.

I take the following excerpt from the journal entry I made an hour after my experience. Some of it's what I remember, and some, what others who witnessed it told me.

*"Wow. Got to the top of the mountain where the sacred site was and WOW. I closed my eyes, started the meditation, and completely lost time. Where the trees previously formed a solid canopy in the sky above me, it seemed like they opened, and I felt the warmth and brightness of the sun on my face. It was a bitterly cold day; snow fell not far from where I stood, but I lifted my face up to the warm light and breathed deeply. That is when the wind started— almost a cyclonic wind. I'm sure it wasn't there a moment ago. It was loud and supernatural. It felt like a vortex. Sucking me down into the earth but rising me up into the sky at the same time. The sun so warm on my face felt like a divine intervention keeping me alive. The energy in me and surrounding me pulled and pushed me. I don't know if I was moving or if I was still, but I felt like I was sitting on a giant wave being carried up and down."*

*"It was the most magical experience of my life. At that moment I felt 'chosen', 'huge" 'tall', 'powerful', 'in control', 'calm' and 'at peace.' I arched my body back to feel as much of the light and*

*warmth as I possibly could, but I wasn't afraid of falling backward. I was held and supported by the light and the wind by my vortex."*

*I cried, not from sadness but a feeling of pure love. **I** was love. **I** was joy. **I** was my happiness. I smiled and stopped crying. The surge of the wind grew, then calmed with each surge of emotion. The wind was getting beneath me and lifting me each time I breathed in and placing me delicately down when I breathed out. I wanted to go with the light and the wind then. I never felt so much love and joy. I was so loved. I felt like it asked me if I wanted to go with it and I said, "Yes, please take me."*

*The next moment, I saw my daughters and Toby, and I felt like my heart and throat would burst inside my chest. The wind quietened. The intense light and warmth retreated, and I stilled. I concentrated on my breathing. (I sob as I write this memory to share with you.)*

*I don't know how long after I first closed my eyes, but I became aware of sounds and smells around me. I opened my eyes to see almost everyone had left. Three people remained. The two retreat leaders, one standing about a metre behind me to stop me toppling backwards if I did, and the other standing about a metre in front of me. Beautiful Jenny stood looking at the altar where past meditators had laid their gifts.*

*I'd experienced my very first transcendental meditation. It lasted for a glorious forty-five minutes. I was in love with life, with my family and with myself.*

## Look inside yourself. There it is waiting for you.

On our walk back to the retreat centre, Jenny told me an incredible story. I have adapted it a little to suit the lessons of my book.

*One day many years ago, the Gods called an immediate crisis meeting. As all twelve Gods sat around the large table, the chief God announced that humanity was in peril and therefore the future of humanity in dire straits. People were destroying each other and themselves, and something needed to be done. The chief God decided humanity needed to be punished and called a meeting to enlist the help of the other Gods to determine how they should be punished.*

*"I want to hide their wisdom, and I need your help to decide where we should hide it."*

*One God answered, "I think we need to hide it in the middle of the ocean. Deep down beneath the ocean floor."*

*The chief God considered this carefully. "No, they will design a way to get out to the middle of the ocean. Then they will create a machine that can drill into the ocean floor. They will find it there."*

*The Gods agreed.*

*Another God suggested, "In the desert. If we put it into the hottest desert, we can bury it there. It will be too hot for any human to withstand."*

*The chief God considered this. "They will create a machine to get themselves there and not perish from the heat. Or they will design a machine to do it remotely for them, so that they don't have to be in the desert at all. They can be very clever at navigating things that are outside of themselves."*

*The Gods agreed.*

*A third God tried with, "We can blast it into space. They will never find it there because they don't know the extent of space that exists."*

*The chief God considered this option carefully and with a shake of the head said, "No, that won't work either. They will eventually discover it. They will discover that there is a space sooner or later, and they will want to do what humans do and insist on learning all about it. Then they will design a machine to get into space. No, they will find it if we put it there."*

*The Gods agreed.*

*Silence engulfed the table as the group considered places to hide humanity's wisdom.*

*The chief God rose sharply from the table. "I have it. We will hide it deep within themselves. The humans will never consider looking for it there."*

*All the Gods passionately agreed and, with one movement of their hands, the command was completed.*

> Humankind's wisdom and the secret to their joy was forever buried deep within themselves.

## How to manage the external pressure. How do you talk to yourself?

Take one high achiever and add a need for approval. Mix in some perfectionism, people-pleasing and a need to solve problems. Add people, topped with a huge serving of suspicion and lack of trust with a sizeable dollop of fear of missing out, and you have one tightly bound ball of anxiety.

Throw social media into the mix over the last five years and bang, welcome to the frenzy. Humans are such great storytellers, but if the stories we tell ourselves aren't encouraging and kind, you can't expect to get the best out of ourselves. 'I need to do it better and faster.' 'I need to be fitter, prettier, and stronger.' 'I need to make it look easy while making it to the top of my game.'

I notice my self-talk can be detrimental when I've spent too much time on social media. I once did the following exercise for one day to measure how social media affected my self-talk. Try it yourself for one day.

Exercise - Choose a day, any day. Preferably a day when you know you would typically spend too much time on social media. When scrolling, observe what catches your eye and subsequent self-talk, then do your Mantra and write down your new self-talk. See what happens.

---

**Write down**

**1.** Cause - What you saw.

**2.** Your self-talk - What came into your mind the minute you saw the thing that made you stop scrolling.

**3.** Mantra - Breathe in –"I love myself." Breathe out –"Yes."

**4.** Reworded self-talk - Now that you love yourself, change your self-talk. What would you say to someone you loved if they'd said your self-talk?

---

In the spirit of my book's message of empowerment, below are my examples, but you never have to show yours to anyone. Please don't judge me.

*ONE*

**1.** Cause - Looking at the post of a woman who got up at 4am to exercise.

**2.** Self-talk - *"Why can't I be like that? I have no discipline. I'm so useless."*

**3.** Mantra - Breathe in – "I love myself." Breathe out – "Yes."

**4.** Reworded self-talk - *"I will move my body however feels right for me today. It's still early, and I have ample opportunity to move my body."*

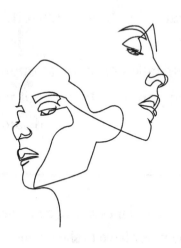

*TWO*

**1.** Cause - Looking at a post by someone gushing over another skincare range. The same person told me only last week her skin had never been so smooth and clear since she started on *my* skincare range one month prior.

**2.** Self-talk – *"What? But they were only saying a few days ago how much they loved my skincare and now they're posting on their Instagram saying how much they love so and so's skincare! What did I do wrong?"*

**3.** Mantra - Breathe in – "I love myself." Breathe out – "Yes."

**4.** Reworded self-talk – *"You haven't done anything wrong. You cannot control other people, what they say or what they do. You can only control how you react to what people say and do."*

THREE

**1.** Cause - Looking at another clinic's Instagram page, the number of followers they have and, in particular, the claim they are experts in cosmetic medicine and treating skin.

**2.** Self-talk - "*Grrrrr. Do they know how many years, twenty years in fact, that I have been studying and perfecting the ingredients for my skincare range? How do they have so many followers? They've been open for two months, and already they have more followers than me. For goodness' sake, they just finished university and have no clinical experience in any area of medicine. Suddenly they know everything about skin and aesthetic medicine. Well, let me tell you, I've looked at the ingredients of your skincare, and there isn't anything in them that will create ANY changes to your patients' skin. I followed therapeutic guidelines for dermatology when creating my range. They wouldn't even know what the therapeutic guidelines are. They have only been looking after skin for twenty minutes, and they think they know what I know. Twenty years, my friend. TWENTY YEARS!! Damn them and damn the person who posted this.*'

**3.** Mantra - Breathe in – "I love myself." Breathe out – "Yes."

**4.** Reworded self-talk – *"Unfollow, unfollow, unfollow. You don't need to feel angry or upset. You cannot control other people, what they say or what they do. You can only control how you react to what people say and do. If their posts trigger you, unfollow."*

*FOUR*

**1.** Cause - Looking at the Instagram page of a clinic that has recently opened. The practitioner did a Bachelor of Nursing and then a quick 2-day course in injectables. She opened the next day in her own clinic. The content on their social media page is all about encouraging young women to have more and more Botox and dermal fillers injected into their faces.

**2.** Self-talk – *"Oh, come on! This is so wrong. The women you're posting on your site are about 12 and you've photoshopped and filtered them like mad. They look terrible with those massive lips, and ridiculous jaws. You're advertising the price of a treatment too, which is illegal. $199 for lips. Come on! What are you using, air? The comments are even more insane. Young women in a frenzy asking for the same treatment. You're responsible for the crisis women are experiencing. You're to blame."*

**3.** Mantra - Breathe in – "I love myself." Breathe out – "Yes."

**4.** Reworded self-talk – *"Unfollow, unfollow, unfollow. You don't need to feel angry or upset. You can't save everyone. Educate your audience. You cannot control other people, what they say or what they do. You can only control how you react to what people say and do. If their posts trigger you, unfollow."*

*FIVE*

**1.** Cause - Looking at the Instagram page of a clinic that has an endless supply of what looks like professionally edited before and after images of patients.

**2.** Self-talk – '*Oh my, how do they get their before and after pics so good? I wish my patients would let me post their before and after pics too. My results are excellent. Why don't they let me post them on social media? Well, I suppose I don't ask them if I can because I don't want them to feel uncomfortable. I couldn't bear it if they said no. That's why I don't post them. Gee, I'm so worried about upsetting people. I am rubbish at this social media stuff, aren't I?*"

**3.** Mantra - Breathe in – "I love myself." Breathe out – "Yes."

**4.** Reworded self-talk – "Breathe. *You aren't rubbish. Your patients love you. You have a completely different focus. You're not interested in posting the big changes in faces. Your specialty is the little changes in your patients' faces. Creating Beautiful Unique Faces. Keep doing this. It's your specialty. That's why you're booked out three months in advance. No one is your competition. If their posts trigger you, unfollow.*"

SIX

**1.** Cause - Looking at the Instagram page of someone I don't even know but seem to be following, who's on holiday with their family.

**2.** Self-talk – *"Oh wow, where are they? On holiday again, I see. Gee, it must be nice to have all that time off. Do they even work? How do other people get all this spare time to enjoy beautiful moments with their children? It's not fair. I'm a terrible mother. I'm a terrible wife."*

**3.** Mantra - Breathe in – "I love myself." Breathe out – "Yes."

**4.** Reworded self-talk – *"If you're feeling unworthy from looking at this post, unfollow, unfollow, unfollow. You know that nothing you see on social media is real. This is a photo of a filtered, heavily directed, and edited moment in time by someone you don't know. Comparison will make you feel bad. You are a wonderful mother and wife. Give your children and husband a cuddle right now."*

## What I do when social media gets me down.

Your Peeps have never seen a post on social media. All they're aware of is your good or bad feelings and the fall out you experience from seeing a post on social media. If you're distressed or feeling self-loathing, so too are your Peeps. But they don't understand why. Think of your Peeps as your babies or people you care about deeply in the world. Would you subject them to the pain and feelings of self-loathing you get from looking at social media? Exactly. Of course, you wouldn't.

I get affected by social media just as much as you do. It drives me insane. I feel depressed that people are living better and happier lives than me. I see women looking better, more rested, more comfortable in their skin than me. I see them having fun with their loving families, being loving mothers and wives AND achieving endlessly in their careers. We forget that it's just the highlight reel, not the full story. If the picture they share tells me they are in some exotic and beautiful location it can send me way down into the depths of despair, just as it does you. Especially if it's with their children and husband and the love is radiating from the photo.

There are bots on your phone and in your computer and in all of your devices that pick up when your scrolling speed slows down. If you slow down on Instagram to look at pictures of an account that brings about feelings of self-loathing, guess what? They will show you more posts not only by this account but of accounts similar to it. They bombard you with the very thing that upsets you the most. My mother always told me when my brothers were teasing me, "Ignore them, and they'll go away." She was right, ignore the pages, the accounts, the people that upset you, and they'll always go away, but hover over them, and you'll be inundated with more and more of the same.

So, what do I do when social media gets me down? Pick any or all of these things to help get you out of your rut.

**If I'm at home and I have a bit of time up my sleeve.**

**1.** Get off my device immediately. I turn it to Airplane Mode and put it away if possible, in my handbag, a drawer. Better still, put it in a drawer in a room, walk out of that room and close the door.

**2.** Take six deep breaths in and out. Box breathe if possible, counting to 4-6 for each breath in, hold, breath out, hold.

---

Exercise: **Box breathing**

Eyes can be open or closed.

If my eyes are open, I look for a wall, a painting, a tree, or if I'm in the shower or bathroom, a tile. I create a box from whatever I am looking at. I breathe in while counting to 4-6 and my eyes trace up the wall, tree, tile, etc. Then I breathe out and trace the width of the object, then I breathe in again and trace down the wall. Last, I breathe out and go back across the width again. This way, I end up back at my starting position, and I repeat the process again 4-6 times.

If my eyes are closed, I imagine the box in my mind's eye and follow the same pattern. Breathe in (trace up), breathe out, (trace across), breathe in (trace down), breathe out (trace back across to my starting point).

---

**3.** Say hi to my Peeps and start with my Inner Power Practice. Observe my Peeps off the back of the box breathing I've just completed. Peeps need movement, and breath is the best way to get them to ride the wave. Check in with my Peeps. Talk to the quiet ones. Ask them how they are. Sit silently breathing and await their response. Tap it out. Tap on whatever my Peeps have told me. See what else comes up from Tapping. And last, I say my Mantra. In breath – "I love myself." Out breath – "Yes."

**4.** Have a big refreshing drink of water in a unique glass. Feel it in my body, cleansing my blood.

**5.** Declutter. I have only recently found the power of decluttering physical objects. I organise something. If I'm at home, I put a load of washing on. The act of washing clothes is hugely therapeutic.

**6.** Clean my bathroom sink. Wipe away the toothpaste and hair that is stuck to the sides. Wipe the benchtop around my sink. Put away the items that don't belong on my bathroom benchtop. I keep a glass cleaning cloth in my bathroom and clean the taps. Clean, shiny taps make me feel so special. Get my favourite hand towel and hang it beautifully in my bathroom.

**7.** Walk around my garden. I sit on the grass, close my eyes, smell the earth, listen to the sounds around me. Take another six breaths in and out. Water my plants.

**8.** Walk into the room and talk to my children. Say hi to them while smiling and looking at them deep in their eyes. Kiss the top of their heads, smell them and tell them I love them.

**9.** Make me and my husband and a cup of tea. Find my husband. Smile at him and say hi. Kiss the top of his head, smell him, and tell him I love him. Drink our tea together.

**10.** Make my bed. Arrange the cushions. Clear the clutter off my bed.

**11.** Make my children's bed and put their favourite toys on their beds.

**12.** Walk around my house. Draw the curtains and open the windows in each room but don't get sucked into the mess of the rooms, I just open the windows and let the fresh air in.

**13.** Decide which is my favourite room in my house at that moment. Stand in the doorway and decide what it is I love most about that room. Clear the clutter from around that thing, make it stand out even more, and stand back and appreciate it.

## If I'm not at home.

It can be more challenging when not at home, but all of these things can be done without anyone even knowing.

**1.** Get off my device immediately. I turn it to Airplane Mode and put it away if possible, in my handbag, a drawer. Better still, put it somewhere discreet and walk away from it.

**2.** Take six deep breaths in and out. Box breathing as described above. You can use your computer monitor to mimic the box for your box breathing.

**3.** Say hi to my Peeps and start with my Inner Power Practice. Observe my Peeps off the back of the box breathing I've just completed. Peeps need movement, and breathing is the best way to get them to ride the wave. Check in with my Peeps. Talk to the quiet ones. Ask them how they are. Sit silently breathing and await their response. Tap it out. Tap on whatever my Peeps have told me. See what else comes up from Tapping. And lastly, I say my Mantra. In breath – "I love myself." Out breath – "Yes."

**4.** Have a big refreshing drink of water. Feel it in my body. Cleansing my blood.

**5.** Stand up and walk somewhere else. Move my body. It doesn't have to be big to attract attention to myself, but it does have to circulate the blood and the stagnant brain chemicals that are trapping my thoughts.

**6.** Leave my phone elsewhere while I walk. Try to get a view of some sky or a vista of some sort out of a window. I appreciate the vista. Look at the shapes of the buildings from the window, the way the light reflects off them.

**7.** Say hi to or smile at someone, and only if I feel like it, engage in conversation with them.

**8.** If I need to, return to the place I left but do not pick up my phone.

**9.** Every time I think about picking up my phone or looking at social media, take six breaths in and out.

The two things I want you to take away from this chapter:

One, social media is not real. Media is not real. All that is real is you right here at this moment right now. You are more than strong enough to walk away from those things that do not serve you or make you feel worthy.

Two, airplane Mode on your smartphone is your best friend.

## Creating healthy boundaries.

You have twenty-four hours in your day. Don't get stuck on wasting any of that time on self-loathing or guilt generating.

**1.** Have your phone or device out of your bedroom. If you use it as you alarm or to play white noise when going to sleep and need it in your bedroom, promise yourself that you'll not look at it after lights are out. Or in the middle of the night or when you first wake up in the morning.

**2.** As soon as you wake, stretch your body in bed. Have you ever seen the utter enjoyment a baby or an animal gets from having a good ol' stretch? It's just beautiful to see. Either stretch your arms above your head or in a wing like fashion to your sides. Stretch your legs out long and stretch and sigh. Observe the wave of ecstasy as they hit your body. The small things in life are often the most delicious.

**3.** Write in your journal. One of the first books I ever read about finding my path was Julia Cameron's *The Artist's Way*. It appealed to me as it focused on creative ways to set you on your journey. *The Artist's Way* recommends writing three pages on waking. Although I regularly fall off this bandwagon, I have found this has been an excellent way to clear my head over the years. In essence, it enables you to get out anything your intelligent brain has processed in the night. If you cannot think of anything to write, write precisely that. "I don't have anything to write today." Fairly soon, your brain will give you something, and it will come out on the page. Even if it's only one sentence, it is exactly what you are meant to put down on paper at that time. Write whatever comes into your brain. Do not edit. Do not worry about neatness. Do not read over. You may even need to write more than three pages. If so, let it all out. Whatever is required in order to a) get your three pages written and b) to set you on your path for the day ahead.

Soon after a close friend was diagnosed with cancer, I sent her a copy of the book, *The Artist's Way*. She got into the habit of writing three pages every morning. She found it was a help during the diagnosis and treatment stages of her illness as she could work through all the stuff in her head that she didn't know how to put into words.

Our brain does vast amounts of problem processing while we sleep. Sometimes we can wake with the answer to something we've been considering for a while. Your three pages will tap into your Peeps and give them an open channel of communication with you. It's important to get our reasoning out on paper as soon as we wake and well before letting our devices or someone else's lives filter in and muddy our minds. If you can, complete your Inner Power Practice immediately after completing your three pages.

**4.** This is a challenge, but try it at least once before judging it as impossible. Pop your phone on Airplane mode and do your morning routine, whatever that may be. Exercise, bathe, eat breakfast, get the family ready and get out the door to work, all *without* looking at social media, reading text messages, messenger messages, Instagram messages or emails. Don't let any of that stuff suck the life out of you in the morning. If anyone needs me urgently, I believe they will call my husband or I and I will not miss out on anything I desperately need to know about. Today, every little thing can be blown up as an urgent thing when it just isn't.

These things **are not urgent** and therefore need to be ignored:

- Any commentary on social media about anything.
- A celebrity or friend fall out that does not directly involve or threaten the safety of you or a member of your immediate family.
- The news. Unless your job is as a journalist, **ignore the news**. I cannot recommend this highly enough. Call me stubborn, but my mental health is much more important than news outlets dramatically informing me of some catastrophe or other that has occurred overnight. The delivery of news is dramatised and sensationalised, I believe, to force us to feel pain and a collective sense of doom. Shocking news headlines, dramatic musical scores underpin news reports like the trailer to a superhero movie. Photographs of grief-stricken people and scenes of carnage, all force us to feel pain and hopelessness. It is all around us. They've taken away our choice when and where we view this stuff. I was at the service station with my husband and children the other morning. As my husband was filling up the car, a giant rolling video screen glared at us, showing the latest news headlines and celebrity dramas.

It's strange to think those in charge of the delivery of news seem hell-bent on sadistically forcing us to see things we just don't want or need to see. Gutter journalism and the sensationalism of trauma, all make us desensitised to bad things. We almost expect the worst, and as a result, go looking for it on our devices and in our lives. News corporations dictate the boundaries, and they're hell-bent on making it harder for us to look away.

**A real catastrophe has already hit our shores, and for many of us, our overworked and frayed coping mechanisms shut down in catatonia.**

## If you need to know about it, someone will tell you.

If there's something you need to know about in the news, you will hear about it, trust me. If you are likely to be directly affected by something, your mother, brother, neighbour, friend, or barista will tell you. Besides that, you do not need to know what rubbish some gutter news company is trying to sell you. The promise of the world imploding and our need to feel helpless and depressed is more often than not a lie. Like the friend who always makes you feel sad and down, by being a Debbie Downer themselves or making you feel anxious and bad about your own life, put them on mute.

Every time I see her, I have a friend who insists on bringing up doom and gloom stories I have shared with her in the past. She especially likes to revisit the stories of people who've upset me. After reliving these stories, she then wants to go in with the killer line of, 'Gee, people have mistreated you.' I always leave our catch-ups feeling down and paranoid that those around me do not respect me and she's right. That I'm always being taken advantage of, which just isn't true. I have made a special effort to reduce our catch-ups, and if she brings up all the bad things that have happened to me in the past, I nip it quickly in the bud and change the subject to something positive and happy.

The problem is, if I turn on my phone and instantly start my day by reading someone's messages to me or posts on a chat, I am immediately involved in that conversation. In one fell swoop, someone has woken me from a deep sleep, opened the door to big brother, and pushed me into a room full of drama. My brain is being pulled in every which way. I am forced to make decisions I don't want to make at that time. Ultimately, the focus has been taken off the sacred routine of getting myself and my family ready for our day. The chance of us having a great day is ripped from us by someone who has no meaning in our lives. And that just isn't fair.

If I look at my emails, I'll inevitably start work, which makes me cranky because, once again, work has infiltrated my family and home life. Being a business owner, I have blurred the line between work and family for almost twelve years. After my burnout in 2019, I decided I needed time well away from work, and that means no work in family and home time. My husband has taken over doing all the business management and financial running of my business. The time this has freed up for me allowed me to write this book. I used to come home from treating in the clinic at the earliest at 7pm.

Having missed out on tea and bath time for my daughters, I would kiss them goodnight and get frustrated when they wanted and needed me to stay with them singing lullabies. I'd stress about the one hundred emails I'd received that day I was yet to open and respond to. On average, I would work until 11pm, fall asleep exhausted with my laptop on my lap, and wake again at 2am with cortisol pumping through my body, telling me to wake up and start work again. I don't know what happens at 2am, but it's like the grim reaper of self-loathing enters my world.

It is so important to set clear boundaries for yourself and those around you. That way, you know exactly when you will be present with your family, your friends, with your me time and with work commitments. Be firm about where family time stops, and work time starts. More importantly, where work time ends, and family life begins.

This has been paramount in my recovery. I can't stress the importance of keeping family time sacred from all forms of interruption, both work and any kind of distraction such as social media, emails, and news. Ask yourself this; if this is not an emergency, is what I am doing right now increasing the love I feel for myself or my family? Ask your Peeps what you need to do right here right now. If it is not nurturing the love for yourself or your family, close it down immediately. Write it on a piece of paper to revisit in work time and let it go. It's not important at all.

Once you start your workday, whether in the office, in your home office, or a cafe, then you start work. Commit your time to opening emails, answering phone calls, and doing your work tasks. Dedicate work time to just that, working. Don't become distracted on your phone. If someone employs you, it isn't fair to them to spend your working time on social media and answer private messages. If you are self-employed, it gives your brain the message that your business isn't legitimate or worthy and can be interrupted by unimportant personal distractions.

I can hear you asking; *"When can I check my Facebook, Instagram, Twitter and Tik Tok accounts? And when can I look at the news?"*

It's an interesting one. It depends on whether social media is part of your work, in which case you need to be on top of it once your work starts and not before. Otherwise, if it's not part of your work, leave it until your 'waiting time.' When you're waiting for your coffee, having your lunch break, are on the train, waiting for your taxi to arrive, or waiting for your business meeting guests to arrive. Whenever you have only a minute here or a minute there, but not when you are supposed to be doing something else productive. Only check social media when you're waiting. It's an easy way to remember. Check social media only when I am waiting. You will be quite surprised how little you need social media, once you understand it's not a need, but a stop-gap to fill the 1-3 minutes you have only when you're waiting.

It's so refreshing not to get sucked into altercations and dramatisations occurring in social media land. I have watched wars of words unfold between people and groups that have sucked the life and energy out of me as an observer. I can only imagine the negative effect it's having on the participant's brain chemicals. If the interaction you're involved in or observing doesn't make you feel good or give you good energy from excitement, get off the device. Your 'waiting time' must surely be over by now, so move on to the next part of your day.

It's our fault we feel like we can't live without our devices. It's not the device's fault and not the fault of the creators of Facebook, Instagram, Twitter, or Tik Tok. It's our fault. Take responsibility for being an adult. If you announce to the world that you're having a digital detox, it will only encourage people to comment, privately message, call and text you, encourage gossip to find out why. It will make your serotonin levels spike and stop you from getting off social media at all. Just leave peacefully. You are closing the door to all the stuff you don't need, quietly behind you. No door slamming tantrums in sight.

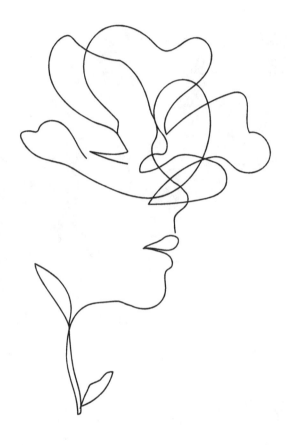

# Chapter Nine

# CELEBRITY PRESSURE.

CASE STUDY: LEAD ACTRESS

## Life on a film set.

*The Director's eyes bulged. "She can't move her face," he hissed.*

The makeup artist closed her eyes and nodded in agreement.

*"We're shooting the death scene. She's meant to be desperate!"*
*He pointed at the camera, "Look! Her face, it's weird," and*
*zoomed in close-up.*

*"Her lips!" He glared and waited for the makeup artist to*
*suggest something. "Can you fix it?"*

*"I can smudge her makeup, like she's been crying...?"*

*Annoyed, he shook his head.*

*"I can't make her face normal again because she's had*
*BOTOX."*

I witnessed this tense interaction between the executive film
director and head makeup artist in the costume department of a

film set in London.

It was 2004, and I had a part in what was a mid-budget film. We shot for six weeks on location.

The lead actress, who was in her mid-thirties, had several essential and emotionally demanding scenes. The audience was to be taken on her heartbreaking journey of loss and then were to witness her rise from the brinks of despair like the phoenix, triumphant at the film's conclusion. It was a dream role for any actress and a brilliant story about the strength of the human spirit.

The problem was that the Botox paralysed her facial muscles and made it impossible to interpret her feelings.

Facial expressions are a global cue for interpretations. Within one second of looking at someone's face, we judge whether that person is safe to approach. Are they happy? Are they sad? Are they angry? Are they open to me approaching them? Based on our interpretation of another's face, we decide if someone is nice or nasty, cranky, or calm. It's an innate human behaviour, and studies show that babies just a few days old can differentiate between a happy or sad face and respond in kind. In short, behaviour breeds behaviour. We mimic emotions as we see them, and we also respond accordingly.

No wonder the sudden injection of Botox before this crucial day's filming devastated the director. The audience would never empathise with and be moved by her story if they couldn't feel, interpret, and mimic her emotions.

I don't know why the lead actress felt compelled to get Botox injected into her facial muscles. Or to double the size of her lips in the lead up to her most challenging and what should have been most acclaimed acting role. I did, however, understand the pressure she must've felt to look perfect. I was devastated for her and also for the film's director. At the time, I was a Princess commencing her raw and messy transition into becoming a Queen. The lead actress was a Queen I admired and aspired to be like. I'd placed her 1-2 steps ahead of me for many years by then. The experience left me reeling with confusion, and I felt betrayed by her.

It was that day on set that began my complex and petrifying journey into the world of Botox, dermal fillers, and cosmetic facial enhancement. I wondered if it was possible to do these things subtly and enhance rather than distort and paralyse the face from these procedures. I also questioned whether in attempting to perfect our face, we were instead diluting our real beauty, our unique facial feature, and inadvertently becoming less beautiful than when we started.

## I'd done something to upset her.

In the weeks after the heated exchange between the director and lead actress, I noticed more women around me, who I suspected had Botox and dermal fillers.

I went to dinner with a good friend, and I noticed her face looked different. Like the actress who couldn't express emotion, my friend's face became distorted when she told a story about something funny or sad. It was hard to gauge what she was feeling from her face. I relied entirely on the words she was using to know what underlying feeling she was expressing and how to respond appropriately.

It was such an uncomfortable dinner. All night I felt she was upset with me. Her typically warm demeanour was frosty and contrite. Eventually, I asked her if I'd upset her in some way.

She seemed surprised and asked why I thought that. I told her she seemed distant and looked different. In explanation, she told me she'd had Botox. She was going for a promotion at work and would be up against some younger women going for the same role.

I understood firsthand the pressure actresses felt about their physical appearance. Given you get shortlisted for the initial audition based purely on a photo of your face, appearance is the most judged part of a female actor. While the pressure on male actors exists too, it is not comparable to how they treat female performers.

The more I considered it, the more I empathised with why the lead actress resorted to Botox to soften lines and wrinkles that possibly made her feel unattractive.

The pressure on all women is to look good all the time. And they magnify the pressure on women who are also actors.

If we examine female actors in their mid-30s versus male actors in their 30s, they overlook women for roles in place of younger actresses. Yet men have a staying power that can see them gainfully employed well into their 50s. The societal pressure on women is to look young and beautiful forever.

Overhearing the conversation between the director and the makeup artist sparked my interest. Yes, while acting and truthfully playing a character had become my life. I was a young woman who was newly single and regularly judged based entirely on my attractiveness in my personal life and my career as an actor and TV presenter.

In 2004, social media wasn't prolific and didn't infiltrate our lives as it does now. Still, amongst my acting circles, I'd heard the lead actress plummeted into depression following the release and subsequent 'flop' of the film we shot. Thankfully, she resurrected her career to a point though and from that day on learned to tread cautiously around the subsequent treatments she received. She sometimes got it just right, enhancing her Unique Facial Feature, her incredibly vulnerable eyes and other times getting it a bit wrong.

## Everybody matters.

Caroline Flack in 2019, Annalise Braakensiek in 2019, Charlotte Dawson in 2014 and too many lost souls who felt they were unworthy, have taken their lives because of the immense pressure they felt when they compared themselves to others. To take your own life is the ultimate act of desperation and agony. In light of the recent deaths of celebrity women and men, who rightly should revel in what their hard work has enabled them to achieve, we need to examine what's going wrong. The minute they set foot in front of a camera, they feel compelled to look and act a certain way. Every part of them scrutinised under a magnifying glass. Even if they are mentally strong before setting out on the first step of their celebrity journey, they're at a much greater risk than you or I of falling prey to what the media and society tells them is beautiful. They feel they need to have perfect features and perfect lives.

You've heard the comment, "celebrities all look the same."

Well, there's an excellent reason for that. The pressure they feel to have the perfect lips, cheeks, chin, and jawline means they all end up ordering the same items off the facial features menu. However, once they achieve this perfected look, they are scrutinised by the media and public alike for either 'overdoing' it or looking 'weird.' The pressure they felt, which led them to have it all done in the first place, intensifies. They can't win! They're damned if they do and damned if they don't. Confusion about why they don't feel better and why the media isn't being kind to them can become too much. It's where the vicious cycle of fill, repeat, fill, repeat begins. Before we know it, the same fresh-faced celebrities we fell in love with at the start of their careers look nothing like they once did. The media and the general public think it's fair game to rip these injured animals to shreds. No one can withstand vast amounts of online abuse and ridicule. It turns previously positive and happy people into self-loathing shells of their former selves, all from being criticised online and in the media.

Who gave the media and every person with a device the right to have an opinion on your life? I have witnessed the vitriol that people sitting behind their screens are willing to dish out. It's disgusting, and it's everywhere. Community groups, celebrity pages, school groups, church groups, political party sites, none are immune to the action of weak and pathetic individuals who think it's ok to speak ill of and to another human being from behind their screen. Shame on all who have behaved in this manner. These people should instead ask for forgiveness from those they've slighted and take a long and hard look at themselves. They are responsible for someone believing they are unworthy.

This is harsh, maybe too harsh, but I feel strongly about trolls. If you can be nasty to someone from behind your computer screen, ask yourself what is missing from your life to make you so bitter. Grow up and work it out. You have the opportunity to rectify what is missing. It's no one's fault but your own.

## I'm not good enough.

We're our own worst critic. I know this. These feelings are still so raw and close to me. Last year I was convinced I wasn't living up to the expectations of being the ideal mother, wife, practitioner, daughter, friend, sister, and entrepreneur. Essentially, the only person who put these unrealistic expectations on me was myself. No one sat there and told me I was a disappointment, and yet I still hit rock bottom.

I am one of the lucky ones. *I* was my own worst critic. The evil trolls were in *my* head, not in the magazines, or on social media making fun of my every move, my every look, my every facial feature. I can only imagine the vitriol that celebrities or anyone in the public eye for that matter endures. It saddens me greatly. As a former actor and TV presenter, I know how unfairly judged I was on my appearance. I compared myself to everyone else. I gauged my worth on someone casting me or not in a role. It seems ironic I'm now in a place where my soul calling in life is to ensure women get their strength from their Unique Facial Feature and internal strength. And not in any way through the judgement of others.

What the camera in a professional production studio and on our smartphone captures is altogether very different from what we look like in the flesh.

Cinematography is an aspect of film and TV production that the average person just doesn't understand. How could you? Unless you've tested for or performed in numerous TV and film productions, you've not seen the work that goes into manipulating the lighting, environment, and camera set up to inform the story. It's a mammoth task and one that requires a high level of skill and experience.

When we look at celebrities, reality TV stars, and influencers onscreen (heck when we look at ourselves or anyone onscreen,) we know none of us look anything like that in the flesh. Seeing a photo or video footage of someone only shows them in 2D. Even 3D movies fall short of realistically replicating seeing someone in the flesh.

Not even taking into account the filters that most people use on Instagram, the camera itself shows faces that aren't accurate. Have you ever seen a photo of yourself and thought, "Gee, I didn't realise I looked like that?" It's because the camera fails to show the subtle nuances of your face. It can even dull down your Unique Facial Feature, meaning your Beautiful Unique Face is lost. Facial features look more pronounced in 2D. This misinterpretation, combined with the fact that everyone has a camera in their hot little hands, has escalated the Pretty Ugly Face epidemic.

Let me describe the vicious cycle: Via social media, celebrities are accessible. This leads to an increase in the pressure they feel to be perfect. Often well-meaning people offer their advice on the celebrity's appearance. In equal measure, the nasty trolls spew their opinion. Celebrities are more exposed to nastiness than the average person, and this pressure makes them feel like every aspect of their life is open to judgement.

Often celebrities, reality TV stars, and influencers are incredibly self-conscious. They are harder on themselves than is healthy. They notice their flaws more, and their adorers and haters furthermore highlight their flaws. To gain approval and to feel good, they have work done, which teaches those who look on that they should have work done, too. The celebrity feels forced to fix every perceived flaw and somehow remain 1-2 steps ahead. It's almost become a race now.

So, the celebrities who, keep in mind, are surrounded by other stars feel the pressure to look perfect, and need to have more done to themselves. I mean golly, they even film themselves having cosmetic injectables. Then the public gets more, too, to keep up. You get the picture. It's a bloodbath. A vicious cycle. None of them are considering their Unique Facial Feature, let alone where they should look to find and nurture their happiness.

Normality is transient, but so too is an overfilled and over-frozen face. Thankfully, those who've had their faces overfilled and over-frozen can get things dissolved and let the Botox wear off. They can enlist the help of a practitioner who knows how to identify and nurture their Unique Facial Feature.

## She left the reality TV show and had all the fillers in her face dissolved.

I love seeing reality TV stars who've had too much done to their poor faces before entering whatever experiment it is, to subsequently have it all dissolved once they leave the experiment. Like a beautiful butterfly emerging from its cocoon.

With no focus on their Unique Facial Feature, it's common for big time celebrities to fall foul to the needle and have it *all* done in the belief that it'll improve their appearance. They have access to the best of the most famous practitioners. If celebrities can make the mistakes instead of us, then we can learn the lessons from them and avoid the same mishaps ourselves.

Think Courteney Cox. She got excited, bought all the candies, and it changed her face. Gone was her Beautiful Unique Face, and here was her overfilled, over-frozen, and quite frankly unusual looking face. Her cheeks so puffed up that her eyes changed shape, their beauty now completely overshadowed. Courteney sadly became alien looking. According to magazines, she saw the light and had her dermal fillers dissolved and let her Botox wear off. Courteney now has subtle work done. Work that allows her

Unique Facial Feature to be the lead actor.

It's a celebrity's Unique Facial Feature that sets them apart and makes us fall in love with them in the first place. Think of Jennifer Grey in 'Dirty Dancing.' Jennifer played Baby beautifully. Cute, but strong. Her age, curls, petite frame, and sincere eyes added to her cuteness. Her lovely strong nose gave her appearance the power and conviction she needed to be the perfect heroine to Patrick Swayze's hero.

After the film, although receiving massive acclaim for her acting and looks, Jennifer had a rhinoplasty. She surgically removed what most considered her Unique Facial Feature. I didn't write a lot about plastic surgery in this book. I don't want to comment on plastic surgery changing young women's faces to chase beauty and perfection. Used for the right reasons, plastic surgery can be wonderful. Yet, you can imagine how damaging surgically removing one's Unique Facial Feature can be.

Jennifer changed her nose, although it was perfect for her. As a result, she's barely worked as an actor again. Suddenly, Jennifer looked like any other young actress with delicate and feminine features. The thing that saw her typecast, her unique nose, was gone, and she lost her appeal with it. It sounds similar to the lead actress in the film I was in, who had extensive Botox and lip fillers leading up to her most challenging role. Why do they do it? Because the pressure from external forces becomes deafening. Actors are in the business of being directed, told what to do, how to act, *and* how to look.

We know it's essential to look to people who are 1-2 steps ahead of us for inspiration. Some actresses have done it beautifully well. Staying true to their Unique Facial Feature while having excellently placed cosmetic injectable treatments. It can be done.

Here are some of my all-time favourite actresses who've done it well.

Alicia Silverstone looks as lovely now as she did twenty-two years ago. All of her injectables are subtle and don't detract from her playful eyes. Cameron Diaz is an actress who, by her admission, has gone too far but has come back from the deep end. She didn't like the way it made her look and denies having had anymore since. However, I'm sure if Cameron had it placed well and subtly, she'd feel differently about the benefits of injectables, even as an actress in the spotlight. Christie Brinkley is one such celebrity. She has mastered the balance of well-placed injectables. Singing the benefit of remaining true to your Unique Facial Feature, Christie knows the only way forward is using small amounts and not changing the way you look.

Sharon Stone is one of my all-time favourite actresses. She's a great advertisement for cosmetic injectables done beautifully. Sharon is a strong advocate for knowing what makes you unique and sticking to what brings out the best of you. Perplexed by women who want to have the same features as the next woman. Sharon said, *"There are 400,000 girls with the same nose, gigantic lips... Are they really prettier?"* Sharon is a true Queen.

Congratulations to Natalie Portman, Amelia Heinle, Carla Gugino, Catherine Zeta Jones, Connie Nielsen, Gabrielle Anwar, Gabrielle Union, Jennifer Connelly, Julia Roberts, Kate Winslet, Lena Headey, Natascha McElhone, Penelope Cruz, Salma Hayek, Sandra Bullock and Uma Thurman who, in the quest to look good, have all maintained their Beautiful Unique Faces.

I have treated celebrities, reality TV stars, and influencers in my clinic. My objective with them is no different to my aim with all of my patients—always under-treat and under-correct, and forever remain true to their Unique Facial Feature. The camera picks up the things that can't always be seen in real life. Capturing intimately the instant a face looks unusual because it doesn't move in the way it should, can destroy the actor's portrayal of the character for the remainder of the film or series.

I recently had the pleasure of looking after a delightful woman, who I now consider a friend. They'd selected Angie Kent to be the Australian Bachelorette in 2019. For Angie, we performed the most subtle treatments before she began filming. Never losing sight of her Unique Facial Feature, which is her knock out smile. Angie has the kind of smile that warms your cockles and melts your soul. Authentic beauty and a pure heart. Angie has integrity and depth and kindness in spades. Her smile is the link that creates a connection.

A genuine interest in life, love, and those around her, they chose Angie for her role to be the Bachelorette thanks to her kinship with normal women. Audiences were tired of seeing overfilled and over-frozen faces on TV and longed for someone with whom they could truly connect. Someone to look up to, someone by whom they felt inspired, someone to fall in love with.

You could say Angie was a muse of mine during the writing of this book, and I'm forever grateful for the trust she placed in me, to keep her connection with her audience alive. Although I knew Angie, the rest of the nation didn't. To see them fall in love with her Beautiful Unique Face during the airing of the Bachelorette was the confirmation needed for the importance of the Unique Facial Feature. I am forever proud of how natural Angie looked in the Bachelorette.

Angie is incredibly self-aware and has done a lot of work on her Inner Power Practice and her mindset. She knows more than anyone that to be kind to others, you must first be kind to yourself.

Whenever you feel disillusioned with the celebrities who have succumbed to overfilled and over-frozen faces, look for the stars who haven't. The ones who stay true to their Beautiful Unique Face as a way of maintaining the connection with their audiences. Look to them instead of becoming disheartened by the women who have lost their way. The most we can do for them is hope that they'll find their way back to their lighthouse, their Unique Facial Feature.

Never become so disillusioned by a celebrity, reality TV star, or influencer's face you feel compelled to make a negative comment about them or their appearance. It's cruel and heartless. You wouldn't like it to be said to you, so don't ever be tempted to say it to another. Your nasty comment may be just the thing to tip them over the edge, to be the final straw that alters their brain chemicals once and for all. I beg you, don't be that person!

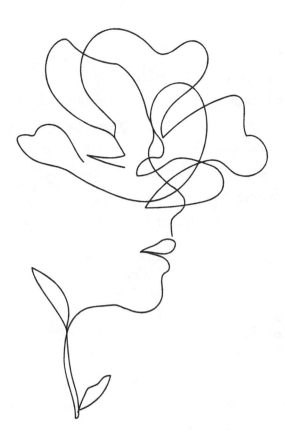

# Chapter Ten

## Part One

# AVOIDING OBSESSION.

CASE STUDY: AMANDA

I remember one of my very first patients with body dysmorphia. It was in 2009, an era before social media was the mainstay. Amanda was a kind, professional, intelligent, and well-presented woman in her early forties. Convinced she was losing volume in her cheeks at an alarming rate, she sought my expert advice. My diagnosis was she'd been over-treated and now had over-inflated cheeks. She'd been told by a practitioner that she had flat cheeks. Subsequently she had approximately 10mls injected in each cheek over the last two years, and in my clinical judgement, this was an excessive amount.

Amanda scheduled in weekly appointments and, when quizzed by reception staff why she needed such regular treatments, she replied they were for different procedures. However, each Friday, she came with the same request, "My cheeks need to be filled," and repeatedly, I asked her to show me where her cheeks had become flat from the previous week. Amanda would look in the mirror and point to imaginary flat spots. I'd reply I couldn't see any flat areas, and I felt her cheeks were already voluminous and didn't need further filling.

Amanda would walk around my treatment room, searching in the handheld mirror and blaming the lighting for failing to highlight where her cheeks had flattened. The flatness was glaringly obvious to Amanda, but not to me. Every week I examined her face, and empathetically told her, "I can only treat what I can see. If I can't see where your cheeks are flat, I can't treat them."

Over her next few appointments, Amanda became increasingly frustrated with me for not being able to see her "flat cheeks." I empathised with her, but continued to refuse to treat her and requested we stretch out her next appointment to six months rather than the following week. I talked to Amanda about body dysmorphia, what it meant, and how it felt to have it. She agreed she spent an above-average amount of time staring at her flaws in the mirror, but denied it negatively affected her.

I offered to refer Amanda to a psychologist and also asked her to visit her GP for advice. She refused and told me she could just as easily go elsewhere for treatment. I agreed this was true and that other clinicians might have less regard for her mental welfare and would happily treat her. I explained why this wasn't ideal for her.

Amanda never returned. I learned she successfully sought and was given dermal filler in her cheeks by another clinician who operated nearby. Amanda was obsessed with her cheeks and in achieving an impossible version of them. She felt a high every time she had them filled.

## Open your mind to possibility.

Harking back to the mountaintop in Italy in 2019, I learned then that we're connected to something immensely powerful, that adores us without question. The answer to our happiness lies within us.

As a spiritual person, I've done a considerable amount of soul searching since that day. This soul searching is what's facilitated the writing of this book. It was the constant striving for betterment and happiness that ironically saw me incredibly unhappy. It's the same struggle that I see in my patients and makes happiness impossible for them too.

We are something, yes, but more than that, we are nothing. We are an empty vessel of nothingness that is most content when allowed to let be and receive what comes to it, wholly and without judgement. When our expectation of ourselves, our life, those around us, and every single thing is nothing, watch the love freely flow. Open your heart to a situation, and the universe will reward you with abundant love. Strive, push, hustle, work harder than everyone else, experience FOMO and envy, and watch the world give you more opportunity to feel this way. Feel unworthy when looking at social media and watch the world give you more of the same. Find endless fault with your face, your body, and your life, but be warned that a tidal wave of the same self-loathing is coming your way. But sit and be nothing but love and watch the world reward you with more of it.

On that mountaintop in Italy, I lost all sense of time, and the space around me became expansive. I was immense; my sense of love was enormous, my connection with the universe was tremendous. The vortex that enveloped me was pure energy. All of my cells sizzled with incredible energy, but not one part of me felt anxious.

Time was endless. I'd all the time I needed. There were no alerts, no reminders, no sensation of having not achieved enough. I was accomplishing exactly what I needed at that moment of my life—my unbridled passion for the universe, Mother Earth, and my existence within her.

When I returned home from my retreat in Italy, I fell hard. Back in my world, which hadn't changed, and unable to recreate the Zen I'd experienced in Italy, I faced the pressure of making, providing, striving, improving, and smashing. I became obsessed with my failures. Failure to mother, failure to wife, failure to daughter, sister, and friend. Failure to make my patients happy.

The chemicals my brain released when I was reminded of my failings became addictive, and I searched for more ways to prove the hypothesis I was a failure. Even when giving up on life, it's incredible how we still want to be right about stuff. I was right. The 2am Monster of Failure that visited me nightly was the biggest cheerleader of my failure. In it, I thought I had a friend and an ally. Regardless of how much my husband, children, and those who loved me tried to tell me I was wrong and that I wasn't failing, the 2am Monster of Failure agreed with me. It enthusiastically played the showreel of evidence for me to watch every morning at 2am.

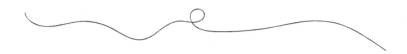

## Part Two

# I AM A RECOVERING DRUG ADDICT.

The knowing I was right about my hypothesis of being a failure gave me the release of dopamine I became addicted to. Searching for evidence on social media and in my life that confirmed the belief about my failings, gave me the brain chemical release I needed, to keep up the drug-seeking behaviour. I have never been a drug user, let alone a drug addict. Still, the brain chemicals, the self-loathing thought pattern makes your brain release, are addictive. In that context, I am a recovering addict.

Too much focus on ourselves is dangerous. We are part of a free, fluid, and never-ending existence. There are no boundaries to where our soul can travel. The connection we feel to the universe is automatically all there. All we need to do is sit and be. There is no work required on our part. It's why the mediation movement has become so necessary. We can't be judged as a good or bad meditator. Everyone's mind wanders. All that is necessary for meditation is that our heart is open, and our mind is still. The mainstay of meditation is the same that grounds us in life, our breath. Meditation creates the opportunity for our heart, soul, mind, and body to connect to expansive space.

I'm a dedicated fan of Dr. Joe Dispenza and Dr. Bruce Lipton. They discuss Quantum Physics, which explains that you are what you think and how you can think yourself into feeling a certain way. It truly is fascinating that we can create all possibility of great things to happen in our life, just as we can manifest the most terrible things, too.

Quantum Physics describes two worlds. The first is the physical reality within which we fight to control every part of our life. We look to create a predictable identity and strive to be something and someone. The second world is the universal or quantum reality, where we lay our faith in the not knowing. We experience joy from not having predictions about how we behave in situations where we have no identity and let surprises come to us.

Classical physics looks at the predictable. When planning scientific experiments, we create a hypothesis of predictability. From a young age, we're controlled by our familiar past and our foreseeable future. Given our brain and body's desire to please, we can almost lay money on the fact that certain things will likely happen to us. Events that have happened to us pave the way for similar events to occur in the future.

If we feel we aren't enough, that there isn't anything beautiful about us or our faces, we will inevitably look for things to confirm it. We can confirm this belief because of social media, body dysmorphia, and an obsession with perceived faults in our face.

Remember the addiction most of us have to the hormone of stress? Well, it reminds us it's the survival of the fittest out there. These chemicals heighten our senses, so we hear, smell, see, feel, and taste more so we can survive. It could even be said they make us 'over sensitive'. Have you ever heard that term? I certainly have. Overreacting to things you shouldn't. The effects of stress mean we feel alone, not connected to anything or anyone. In this physical reality, we're focused purely on the material things we've placed value on.

However, in the universal or quantum field, the less we focus on our identity, the more connection and possibility exist. There is infinite time and space for a myriad of amazing things to happen to, and for, us. If we can't see it, physically touch it and make a plan to acquire it, we have less expectation of it and that it can exist in the true here and now.

> *'Get over yourself.' 'Stop being so narrow-minded.' 'Stop imagining the worst.' 'Build a bridge and get over it.'*

As harsh as these are to hear, they each preach great advice. The more we can stop focusing on ourselves, broaden our focus, and surrender all expectations, the happier we can become.

Stopping our familiar, negative thinking pattern and creating new neural pathways for our water to flow down, allows the sense of imminent possibility. In this space, we are no one and nothing, and this freedom unleashes our true magic.

It feels absurd, doesn't it? We live in a world where everyone is fighting for attention, where every kid gets a prize. Where we judge our worth on the number of followers and likes we get from people we've never met. But the key is to remove yourself from that race. It's a race that no human can win, so save yourself and permit yourself to leave it now.

My one transcendental meditation experience made me feel

at one with the universe. I felt whole, but at the same time, like I didn't exist at all. It's undoubtedly the most freeing feeling I have ever felt. To feel I'm nothing instead of trying to force myself to be something. I crave it.

## Finding your vortex.

While at the time of writing this book, I haven't experienced it again. I can get close enough to smell it by doing these things. If you need to use noise-cancelling earplugs or headphones, be my guest. I get distracted by every little sound. Often convinced I can hear my children screaming out for me when they aren't. If we can linger in a feeling that connects us to the universal field, then we are nourishing our brains and bodies with space to allow love and possibility.

**1.** Get grounded. Bare feet on Mother Earth. Feel the connection of Mother Earth supporting my body and opening my heart. I sense my heart opening like a lotus flower. I place my right hand over my heart space and my left hand on my lower stomach. Feel the abundance of love your body produces. Deep breathe.

**2.** Feel immense gratitude for my beautiful body, the beautiful air I breathe, and the beautiful ground I feel beneath my feet. Deep breathe.

**3.** Check in with my Peeps. Send love to them. Thank them. Deep breathe.

4. Breathing Mantra. In breath – "I love myself." Out breath – "Yes."

**5.** Shift my focus to the space in between my eyes and just in front of my face. We call this the third eye space. This is the space that became my entry to the vortex in my transcendental meditation experience in Italy. It opened the universe to me.

**6.** Now I just sit with my focus on my third eye. I feel love. I feel gratitude. I breathe. The longer I can linger here, in this place, the better. If I get distracted by a thought, a feeling, or a sound or smell, I tell myself, "it's ok" and place my focus back onto my third eye.

And that, lovely people, is it! One minute or one hour? However long you can dedicate to doing this, is wonderful.

If I've meditated in the morning and something in my day sparks those familiar feelings of anxiety, panic, and stress, I imagine myself hovering back in that beautiful third eye space and breathe. If I can do this, I can stop the comfortable but damaging brain pathways in their tracks. The familiar past and predictable future are now less so. The now is unknown. The future is mine for the taking. Life is beautiful, and I am grateful.

## Obsession and where it comes from.

I believe we're all, to an extent today, addicted to stress. The adrenaline our cells produce creates energy in our cells. Enough so our brain perceives the stressor to be huge. This energy we create in an emergency is given to us so we can fight, run, or hide. Today, when we look at social media and compare ourselves to others, it releases the chemicals of stress. When we decide we aren't 'good enough' and are 'unworthy'. When we judge we aren't pretty enough, we release the stress hormones. But instead of running away from a tiger, fighting a burglar, or hiding from a gang who are threatening our family, the threat is in our head and can follow us around continuously.

Your brain cleverly produces seven main chemicals. Each has a unique role in your life. When you chase the right chemical for the wrong reasons, you get into a bad pattern. Obsession and addiction happen when you try to control how your brain releases these chemicals instead of releasing them naturally.

We have four positive brain chemicals and three harmful brain chemicals that are useful when utilised correctly. You could say our brain is hard-wired for seeking pleasure. Our positive brain chemicals are dopamine, serotonin, oxytocin, and endorphins. Our harmful brain chemicals are adrenaline, norepinephrine, and cortisol.

**1. Dopamine** - gives us a sense of receiving a reward. It's the chemical of motivation.

Unhealthy ways our brain releases dopamine:

The ding on our phone telling us that we've received a notification. A like, a follower, a comment on our Instagram post. Caffeine, nicotine, high fat, and high-sugar foods.

Healthy ways our brain releases dopamine:

Meditation, exercise, getting a massage, holding the hand of someone we love, cuddling someone, eating a balanced and healthy diet full of Tyrosine or achieving a task every day.

When you've checked your phone and have seen that someone has commented on your post, your picture, your video, your brain releases dopamine and makes you feel good as a way to reward you. But soon after, that dopamine decreases, and your brain hunts down the next dopamine hit. This is where you need to take control. Only allow notifications for a particular thing. For example, if working, turn off all personal notifications. If relaxing, turn off all work-related notifications. Turn off the notifications for messages you don't need to know about. Only then can you move on. You are in control of what you let into your life.

**2. Serotonin** - is the peer acceptance and the social brain chemical. It's what controls our mood. It gets released when we feel the love and acceptance of ourselves from others. Most antidepressants on the market increase the serotonin level available in our brain.

Unhealthy ways our brain releases serotonin:

Serotonin is probably the most dangerous chemical where social media is concerned. Every one of us is guilty of this. If we receive a positive comment on the photo of our heavily filtered face, it reinforces this behaviour, and we do more of it. Whether that's a video of us getting our lips done, or our lips after they've been filled up again. We make decisions based on what others will think of us, rather than what we want and need.

If we no longer get serotonin from doing good things and achieving accolades, the serotonin hit from social media is short-lived. The guilt we feel afterward is like a bad hangover. The next thing we know, we seek that serotonin hit again, by doing more extreme things to our face. Photoshopping ourselves even more. The bar is placed forever higher, and we'll try anything to get that hit. It's obsessive and addictive behaviour.

Healthy ways our brain releases serotonin:

Eating good healthy food, getting rest, deep breathing, enjoying our hobbies, and reading, singing, dancing, exercising, and cooking.

Do the things that naturally lift your mood. The things that make *you* feel good. Do whatever you like to do. That will boost your mood and your serotonin levels.

Find a different way to get your serotonin rather than relying on peer acceptance. You may fool other people, but you can never really fool yourself. Influencers might tell you they're so happy using whatever product they are endorsing. Still, if they don't believe it, they feel dishonest and hate themselves. The more you attempt this kind of serotonin hit, the more you end up having to do it over again. The comedown yucky feeling from the lie simply makes you hungry for another hit. Share things on social media that genuinely move you forward, but don't post photos of yourself only for the likes. Have a healthy and real social life rather than an apparently-healthy-but-actually-fake social media life. Share things that make you feel good. Join a good cause.

**3. Oxytocin** - The love chemical. This chemical is released naturally when a woman gives birth and, in both parents, when nurturing a child. While oxytocin is the chemical of love and strengthens the bonds you have with your loved ones and your tribe; as a result, it can make you prejudiced against those not in your tribe.

When oxytocin is high, so are the lengths to which you will go to protect those you love, including lying and fighting. Imagine two rival sporting teams. Team A and Team B. The fans of both teams feel comradeship together and against the rival team. They each release oxytocin, meaning they support their team like they are protecting their family. They are fighting the battle together and against their common enemy, the rival team. Wars have started because of the oxytocin.

Unhealthy ways our brain releases oxytocin:

Excluding people who don't have the same ideas as us. In social media we will sometimes feel safe to express prejudice against people with a different opinion or belief than us. Trolls and keyboard warriors are passionate people who act on the release of oxytocin, telling them to protect their people and their belief at all costs.

Healthy ways our brain releases oxytocin:

Getting outside, meditation, watching a funny movie, cuddling a loved one, having a massage, doing something lovely for someone, patting a pet. These are all great ways to gain a healthily release of oxytocin and have the bonus of creating a positive effect on your life.

**4. Endorphins -** are our natural anaesthetic. They reduce the reception of pain in our body. We all know exercise is the best way to release endorphins. Still, as with all things, we have discovered unhealthy ways to release endorphins, too.

Unhealthy ways our brain releases endorphins:

Hyper-focusing on a problem, annoying customer, negative friend, troublesome colleague, or feuding family member. In other words, creating drama where drama didn't exist before.

Chasing drama has become a common phenomenon with the rise and acceptance of social media. People enjoy it. Watching the drama unfold on social media is voyeuristic, and it makes you feel sick. This isn't the movies, though; this is real life, and this stuff destroys lives. Getting involved in, creating, or watching drama on social media releases endorphins, yes, but not the right way. The things people feel comfortable to say on social media, they'd rarely be willing to say to someone's face.

Live by this motto: if what you'll say isn't true, kind, necessary or helpful, keep your mouth zipped up and say nothing.

**https://www.brainyquote.com/quotes/bernard_ meltzer_15751119/4/2020**

Better still, unfollow, turn off all notifications and walk away from the drama. I've unfollowed many groups because of the nasty things people say in them. Choose Kind is the movement born from R. J. Palacio's 2012 novel *'Wonder,'* in which she facilitates the idea that *'choosing kind will inspire a chain reaction of goodwill towards others.'* **https://global.penguinrandomhouse. com/tag/choose-kind/19/4/2020**

Healthy ways our brain releases endorphins:

Exercise, of course. Good healthy exercise, suitable for our individual body and level of fitness. You can also challenge yourself by learning a new skill or playing a board game.

Our three harmful brain chemicals, adrenaline, norepinephrine and cortisol, all do the same thing: prepare you for danger. They redirect the blood utilised for other bodily functions (such as our digestion) to be moved to our brain for increased alertness, large skeletal muscles, and lungs so we can run or fight. And they send blood to our heart, so our blood pressure is nice and high.

Our sympathetic nervous system is stimulated by adrenaline, norepinephrine and cortisol. It's a beneficial and intelligent process our body performs. However, if danger is perceived as being constant, we can have a constant and slow drip of cortisol in our bloodstream and this is very unhelpful. This can be in the form of someone or something in our life or even pressure from social media. No one can live in a constant state of fear. Our parasympathetic nervous system, which is the opposite of the sympathetic nervous system, can't stabilise and relax your body if a slow drip-feed of cortisol is always present. Soon enough, we're addicted to stress.

Every thought we have is biased towards misinterpreting situations to make them worse than they are. The long-term effects of stress cause decreased immunity and disease. Chronic stress stops us feeling connected to ourselves and others. It sees us trying to control every part of ours and others lives. It can make us suspicious, jealous, aggressive, unhappy and over-reactive. And it's at this point where women who try to perfect every facial feature become unstuck.

Continually striving for perfection sees women create a plan for achieving the thing they think will make them look perfect. When it fails to make them happy, they move onto the next thing and then the next and then the next. Soon enough, they have developed depression, anxiety, and body dysmorphia. They believe that happiness comes from a syringe rather than what is inside them. It's the reason I've written this book. The increasing number of women I see in my clinic asking me to make them happy by injecting their faces and giving them perfect facial features breaks my heart.

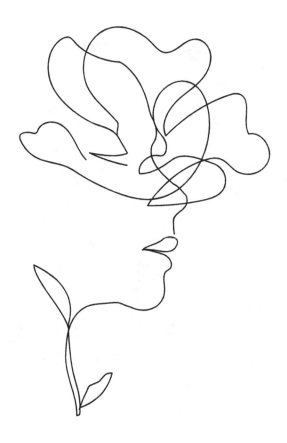

# Chapter Eleven

# FINAL STATEMENT.
# IT'S NOT EASY, BUT IT *IS* SIMPLE.

You have now learned all about the power of your *Inner Power Practice*. You have your one *LIGHTHOUSE* - your Unique Facial Feature, which will guide your every decision when it comes to your face. And you have three *ANCHORS* that will secure you throughout your life, and in every situation you encounter. *Peeps*, *Tapping*, and *Mantra*.

You must take away from reading my book, one overarching belief: This process may not be easy, but it is simple.

In this final chapter I'll summarise everything we've discussed and learned together throughout the book. Easy-to-digest, bite-sized chunks of information you can easily remember and apply to every aspect of your life.

My expertise is the skin and cosmetic medicine and the lessons I have learned over the years with my patients. It is those lessons I have put down on paper so that together, we can all learn how to discover, embrace, accept, and celebrate our uniquely beautiful selves.

With open hearts, we move forward. Away from perfection, the number one enemy of our happiness, and into vulnerability. The discovery of our Unique Facial Feature will lead us to a place of love and joy.

Stop looking externally for validation; there is none to be found there. It's not in the newly injected lips that we see on an influencer's Instagram post, or from the posts we put up of our freshly injected lips either. The vulnerable women who have become Pretty Ugly Faces are not happy, and neither can we be in becoming like them. They need our love and care more than anything now. The validation we receive from social media likes is short-lived. Like a drug, it's addictive and dangerous. The dopamine and serotonin hits we get from the comments last momentarily, and then we feel empty and want more. Recognise this pattern and get dopamine and serotonin from healthy means such as those discussed in Chapter Ten and your Inner Power Practice.

## Stop looking outside for what is already inside you.

**1.** Focus on your **Unique Facial Feature** if and when choosing a **clinic**, a **practitioner**, and deciding on what **treatment** to have done. If the clinic, practitioner, and treatment are concerned with having lots of treatments you don't need, are in 'vogue' on Instagram or the focus isn't about enhancing your UNIQUE FACIAL FEATURE, then do this - Use your legs to do the talking and run a mile. As with every profession, there are unscrupulous operators whose goal is to take your money.

**2.** Talk to and listen to your **Peeps**. A lot. All the time. The Gods buried your wise Peeps inside you. They are your ultimate love. Let them guide you. Let them love you. When you're happy, talk to them. When you're sad, talk to them. When you wake at night, speak with them. Get to know them as you would a new partner. Check in with them. Talk to the quiet ones. Ask them how they are and what they are feeling. Then sit silently and listen.

**3. Tap it out**. Tap about what your Peeps have told you. Tap about everything, anything, and nothing. You can do it discreetly in a group of people, or you can give it your all and tap it out in the shower, so if need be, your tears can flow freely. Notice how I gave you options in that last sentence? You need to tap everywhere and in every situation that calls for it. Tap and see what else comes up.

---

Your basic Tapping script is:

*"Even though I am…, I deeply and completely love and accept myself."*

*"Even though I feel…, I deeply and completely love and accept myself."*

*"Even though no one…, I deeply and completely love and accept myself."*

*"Even though everyone…, I deeply and completely love and accept myself."*

---

There are hundreds of scripts you can find and follow, but I prefer to write my own. My Unique Facial Feature is my Unique Facial Feature, and no one else's. My Peeps will always guide my Tapping script, and yours will guide you too.

Drink water after you finish your Tapping.

**4. Mantra.** Breathe in – "I love myself." Breathe out – "Yes." And repeat how many times feels nice for you. It might be one; it might be one hundred. Your body will tell you when you've reached the point when it's time to stop.

**5. Breathe**. Find your third eye and hover joyously there. See the space that broadening your focus on nothing and no one, gifts you. Remove from your mind all of your ideas about who or what you are. There is no familiar past; there is no predictable future. You are in a time of infinite possibility. Linger with the sense of being nothing throughout your day.

Recognise when you feel:
Anxious
Ugly
Unworthy
Self-hate

Step away from the phone, person, or thought. Instead of reacting, breathe in and out six times and ask your Peeps for help, do a few rounds of Tapping, say your "I love myself" Mantra and look to your third eye.

**6. Beautiful World**
Get your feet on the ground and see, feel, listen, and smell. Get amongst nature, look out a window at a vista of some sort. Look at something like a piece of artwork. Doodle or write out everything that is in your head. Take your focus out of your head and away from the thing that has made you feel anxious internally and onto something amazing in the external world. Lift your eyes from your phone, computer, or device screen, and look up and out. Step

away from your device and enjoy the world.

## 7. Move your body.

Take the stairs. Go to the bathroom that's further away. Park the car further away and walk further. Even run some of the way. Swim or do doggy paddle when in water. Do yoga. Do more yoga and do even more yoga. Do more Yin yoga than Yang. And when your body is feeling less drunk on adrenaline, do Yang yoga again.

## 8. Meditate.

Still your brain and heart through meditation. Change your brain's worry and anxiety patterns. Get dopamine and serotonin release from meditation. There are so many free meditation programs you can download. I love 'Inside Timer' for free mediation courses, Headspace, FMTV, and Gaia for paid courses. Read, listen to, and immerse yourself in Dr. Joe Dispenza and Dr. Bruce Lipton.

## 9. Drink a big glass of water.

You have the cleverest body in the world. Along with your Peeps, your body wants you to be the best it can be. Give it water as often as you can. Your body loves to be cleansed.

## 10. Unfollow all the people.

Restrict, block, unfollow, or unfriend all the people who don't make you feel good about yourself. You do not need that stuff in your life. You have one responsibility; to be kind to yourself so that you can be a kind person to others. Great things come once you treat yourself with love and kindness. If someone or something makes you want to be unkind to yourself, get rid of it. You'd give the same advice to your child or friend if someone or something made them feel self-hate. Be your own protector.

## 11. See a Naturopath.

I am a strong advocate of natural medicine. When I was a teenager, and the root cause of an illness a mystery, my mother took me to see Nancy, our family naturopath. Nancy sorted me out in no time. Never be afraid to examine what you put in your body and adjust it, so that you allow yourself to feel great. Nutritious wholesome food is a change you can make instantly. Limit your alcohol, saturated fats and sugar intake.

Educate yourself on the ways that best heal your body. Western and Eastern medicine have merits of equal calibre. Invest in both.

**12.** Consult your **GP.**

Get your blood levels checked. Hormone, vitamin, and mineral imbalances can play havoc with your ability to think clearly and decipher what's important from what's not. Any niggles you've put off having investigated, seek help for them now. Remember if it's on your mind, it's there for a reason. Confirm or deny it by getting it investigated.

I believe so strongly in you and know that now you're at this point, you have all you need to bid me farewell. With this knowledge you know what is unique about your face. You and all the women around you have Beautiful Unique Faces. I am ready to lovingly kiss you on the head and proudly remove the last bandage from your damaged wing. You're now ready to fly free and be brilliant.

As the phoenix rises from the flames, healthier and more amazing than before, now you, too, are the strongest, most calm and most beautiful you've ever been. You have found your unique wisdom not in something outside of yourself but buried deep within you; your Peeps. You have vulnerably met and fallen in love with your Peeps. A once unrequited love, but now the deepest, most respectful love grows between you both. Your Peeps have your back, and your front and *all* of you. Now you're living. Now you're loving. Now you've arrived.

**Congratulations.**
**I believe in you.**
**I love you.**

THE END

# WORKSHEETS AND EXTRAS

The internal work is yours to enjoy for the rest of your precious life.

The printable worksheets and reminders I have created for you can be found on my website.

**https://www.anitaeast.com.au/books/beautiful-unique-ces-resources/**

Please use these as and when you feel you need a little refresher. Please know that these worksheets and extras are all protected by copyright and therefore cannot be printed and distributed without my personal consent.

# ACKNOWLEDGEMENTS

I have some wonderful people I want to show my gratitude for in the creation of this book.

Toby, the most beautiful husband to me and the most incredible father to Agatha and Daisy. Without you, this book would still very much be a pipe dream. You believed in the power of my book to protect our two darling daughters and motivated me daily, to ensure my words flowed. Thank you for supporting this strong woman.

Agatha and Daisy, thank you for choosing me to be your Mummy. You are the inspiration for this book. You make me a better person every day. Two incredibly strong girls, I love you so very much.

Anjanette, thank you for being the most incredible birth partner for this book. Your love and faith in me during its conception, creation and messy birth, have been invaluable.

Thank you to my awesome family for being my best friends and cheerleaders.

Thank you to Karen for the power of your knowing the

importance of my message. Louisa, for being such a wise and kind editor. Denise DT, for the wonder that is tapping and anchoring.

My awesome Anita East Medispa team, thank you letting me frantically write between patients, and at every spare opportunity.

And ultimately, thank you to all the women I have met in my life. Without you I would never have known how important the message of my book was to spread. May you all relish in your Beautiful and Unique Faces, now and forever.

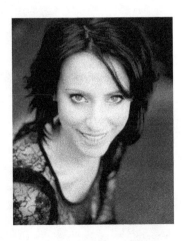

# ABOUT THE AUTHOR

Anita East is the CEO of Anita East Medispa, a clinic specialising in non-surgical cosmetic medicine. She has performed more than 18,000 treatments on people worldwide. A resident writer for The Cosmetic Surgery Magazine,

Anita is often called upon to present at meetings on Cosmetic Medicine throughout Australia an internationally. She is a Nurse Practitioner specialising in skin and cosmetic medicine and holds a BSc, MA and MSN.
Full time mother to two darling daughters, Anita is determined to make the world a safer and more accepting place for when they grow up and ask; "Am I beautiful enough?"

Anita worked as a TV Presenter for Sky Sports, the BBC and UK breakfast television, acted on The Bill, Neighbours, Offspring and Rush, and performed in various TV commercials and films as well as West End theatre shows. Educatin people through storytelling is her passion.

CPSIA information can be obtained
at www.ICGtesting.com
Printed in the USA
JSHW032252150321
12549JS00004B/7